Intermittent Fasting Unleashed
The Mind-Body-Spirit Detox Program

Scott Anthony

WISEGUY
MEDIA

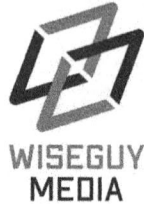

For more information, contact : Wiseguy Media

http://www.wiseguymediapublication.com

Cover design by Boxless Designs

Library of Congress Control Number: 2023920020

ISBN - Paperback: 979-8-9892846-4-1

First Edition: November 2023

Table of Contents

Introduction

In my journey to better health and wellness, I struggled with the challenges of weight loss and the search for balance in my life. Through years of trial and error, I discovered that being truly healthy is more than just shedding pounds – it's about finding harmony among our mind, body, and spirit. This book, "Intermittent Fasting Unleashed: The Mind-Body-Spirit Detox Program," is the culmination of my experiences and the valuable lessons I've learned along the way.

Having realized that everything in our lives connects when it comes to our overall well-being, I knew that if any one aspect were out of balance, the others would suffer. An imbalance often reveals itself through our health, and that's why it's crucial to address all three components – the mind, body, and spirit – simultaneously.

In this book, I hope you'll find a formula for success; a formula that I've crafted through years of personal experience. This isn't just another quick-fix gimmick or fad diet plan – instead, it's a comprehensive program designed to help you create your own plan using small, simple steps towards achieving optimal health.

One key step in this process is detoxification: eliminating those things in our lives that contribute to poor health. By removing toxic influences from our environment and focusing on our ultimate goal of well-being, we can pave the way for a happier and healthier future.

But success doesn't come from implementing drastic changes overnight. The secret to long-lasting change lies in taking small steps consistently over time, which lead to sustainable improvements in both physical and emotional health.

"Intermittent Fasting Unleashed: The Mind-Body-Spirit Detox Program" will guide you through these small steps towards building an effective personal plan tailored to your unique needs. As you journey through this book, you'll come to understand that health encompasses more than just weight loss—it's about finding balance in your life through the perfect blend of mind, body, and spirit nourishment.

Let's take this journey together and unleash our full potential for living our healthiest and most fulfilling lives.

Chapter 1:
The Holistic Approach

In recent times, there has been a growing acknowledgment of the significance of a comprehensive approach to well-being. This perspective recognizes that well-being encompasses not only the absence of disease but a state of complete physical, mental, and social health. In this chapter, we will delve into the fundamental principles of this holistic approach, exploring the intricate interplay between the mind, body, and spirit. We will also introduce intermittent fasting as a tool to enhance holistic well-being.

Defining the Holistic Approach to Well-Being

The holistic approach to well-being is a multifaceted viewpoint that considers the entirety of an individual, covering physical, mental, emotional, and spiritual aspects. It acknowledges that these dimensions are interconnected and interdependent, and achieving genuine well-being requires addressing all of them.

Physical Health:

Physical health is a foundational aspect of the holistic approach to well-being. It encompasses the body's functioning and its overall state of wellness. Several key factors contribute to physical health, and understanding and addressing them are essential for achieving and maintaining a state of optimal well-being.

Nutrition plays a pivotal role in physical health. A balanced and nourishing diet provides the body with the essential nutrients it needs to function correctly. These nutrients include vitamins, minerals, proteins, carbohydrates, and fats, all of which serve various critical functions in the body. Proper nutrition supports growth, repairs tissues, and provides energy for daily activities. It also helps the body maintain a healthy weight and reduces the risk of nutrition-related diseases, such as obesity, diabetes, and heart disease.

Regular physical activity is another cornerstone of physical health. Exercise not only strengthens muscles and improves cardiovascular health but also has a significant impact on mental and emotional well-being. It releases endorphins, which are natural mood lifters, and reduces stress hormones like cortisol. Exercise can enhance flexibility, balance, and overall mobility, contributing to an improved quality of life. Additionally, it aids in weight management and reduces the risk of chronic diseases such as hypertension and osteoporosis.

Sleep is a vital component of physical health and overall well-being. During sleep, the body undergoes essential processes, including tissue repair, hormone regulation, and memory consolidation. A consistent and restorative sleep pattern is crucial for maintaining optimal physical health. Sleep deficiency has been linked to a range of health problems, including increased susceptibility to infections, impaired cognitive function, mood disturbances, and an elevated risk of chronic conditions like heart disease and diabetes. Prioritizing good sleep hygiene and ensuring an adequate amount of quality sleep is essential for physical well-being.

Prevention and Management of Physical Illnesses, proactive measures for the prevention and management of physical illnesses are central to the holistic approach to health. This includes regular health check-ups, screenings, and vaccinations to detect and prevent potential health issues. Additionally, having a comprehensive understanding of one's own health risks and taking appropriate steps to mitigate them is crucial. When physical illnesses do occur, a holistic approach involves seeking medical care, adhering to prescribed treatments, and considering the mind-body-spirit connection in the healing process.

Holistic Approach to Physical Health, the holistic approach underscores the interconnectedness of physical health with other dimensions of well-being. It recognizes that physical health is not isolated but influences and is influenced by mental, emotional, social, and spiritual health. For example, stress and emotional well-being can impact physical health, and conversely, physical ailments can affect mental and emotional states. Therefore, the holistic approach encourages individuals to consider all aspects of their health when addressing physical well-being.

Physical health is a foundational element of the holistic approach to well-being. It involves maintaining the body's optimal functioning through proper nutrition, regular exercise, restorative sleep, and the proactive prevention and management of physical illnesses. Recognizing the interconnectedness of physical health with other dimensions of well-being is key to achieving a state of holistic wellness. By nurturing physical health, individuals lay a solid foundation for their overall well-being, allowing them to lead healthier, more fulfilling lives.

Mental Health:

Mental health is a crucial dimension of the holistic approach to well-being, encompassing our cognitive and emotional well-being. It plays a pivotal role in our overall quality of life, affecting how we think, feel, and interact with the world around us.

Cognitive Function refers to our ability to think, reason, learn, and remember. It includes processes such as attention, memory, problem-solving, and decision-making. Optimal cognitive function is essential for daily tasks, creativity, and problem-solving. The holistic approach recognizes that factors like nutrition, sleep, and stress management profoundly influence cognitive function. Therefore, it emphasizes adopting habits that support cognitive well-being, such as maintaining a balanced diet, getting regular exercise, and managing stress.

Emotional Regulation involves the ability to recognize, understand, and manage our emotions effectively. It's normal to experience a wide range of emotions, but the key is to respond to them in a healthy and balanced way. The holistic approach encourages practices like mindfulness and emotional intelligence to enhance emotional regulation. These practices help individuals develop greater self-awareness and the skills needed to navigate their emotions constructively.

Stress Management, Stress is an inevitable part of life, but chronic or unmanaged stress can have adverse effects on mental health. The holistic approach places a strong emphasis on stress management techniques, such as meditation, yoga, deep breathing exercises, and relaxation strategies. These practices help individuals reduce the physiological and psychological impacts of stress, fostering a greater sense of calm and emotional well-being.

Prevention and Treatment of Mental Health Disorders, the holistic approach acknowledges that mental health disorders, such as anxiety, depression, and bipolar disorder, can impact an individual's well-being significantly. It encourages a proactive approach to mental health by promoting awareness of common mental health conditions, reducing stigma, and seeking timely treatment when needed. Treatment options may include therapy, medication, lifestyle modifications, and social support.

Interconnectedness with Physical Health, the holistic approach recognizes the close relationship between mental and physical health. For instance, chronic physical illnesses can contribute to mental health challenges, and vice versa. Addressing physical health concerns can have a positive impact on mental well-being, and nurturing mental health can support physical recovery. This interconnectedness highlights the importance of holistic care that considers both mental and physical dimensions.

Holistic Approach to Mental Health, a holistic approach to mental health involves integrating various aspects of well-being, including physical health, emotional well-being, social connections, and spirituality. It acknowledges that mental health is not isolated but influenced by a complex interplay of factors. Individuals are encouraged to adopt a well-rounded approach to mental health, encompassing self-care, seeking professional help when necessary, maintaining a supportive social network, and exploring spiritual or mindfulness practices that resonate with them.

Mental health is an integral part of the holistic approach to well-being, encompassing cognitive and emotional aspects of our lives. It emphasizes cognitive function, emotional regulation, stress management, and the prevention and treatment of mental health disorders. Recognizing the interconnectedness of mental and physical health, the holistic approach encourages individuals to adopt a comprehensive approach to mental well-being, promoting a healthier and more fulfilling life.

Emotional Health:

Emotional health is a vital dimension of the holistic approach to well-being, focusing on our ability to understand and manage emotions effectively. It encompasses various facets of our emotional well-being, including how we express, cope with, and navigate our feelings.

Understanding emotional health begins with an understanding of one's emotions. This involves recognizing and labeling different emotional states, from joy and love to anger and sadness. Understanding the nuances of emotions enables individuals to respond to them in a more informed and balanced way. Emotional intelligence, or EQ, plays a significant role in this aspect of emotional health.

Expression of emotionally healthy individuals are comfortable expressing their feelings in appropriate ways. They communicate their emotions openly and assertively, which can foster healthy relationships and prevent emotional suppression. Bottling up emotions can lead to stress, tension, and conflicts, making it crucial to express them constructively.

Coping Mechanisms, Emotional health also involves developing healthy coping mechanisms to deal with life's challenges and stressors. These mechanisms may include mindfulness practices, deep breathing exercises, journaling, or seeking support from trusted friends or professionals. The holistic approach encourages individuals to explore various coping strategies and choose those that resonate with their needs and preferences.

Interconnectedness with Mental and Physical Health, Emotional health is closely intertwined with both mental and physical well-being. Unaddressed emotional issues can manifest as physical or psychological symptoms. For example, chronic stress or unresolved grief may contribute to physical health problems like headaches, digestive issues, or even cardiovascular conditions. Emotional health also influences mental well-being, as emotional distress can lead to conditions such as anxiety or depression.

Prevention of Emotional Issues, the holistic approach emphasizes the importance of prevention when it comes to emotional health. This includes recognizing and addressing potential sources of emotional distress early on, seeking professional help when necessary, and proactively engaging in self-care practices. Preventive measures can reduce the risk of emotional issues escalating into more significant mental health challenges.

Holistic Approach to Emotional Health, a holistic approach to emotional health involves integrating emotional well-being into one's overall wellness plan. It recognizes that emotional health is not a standalone dimension but interacts with physical, mental, social, and spiritual aspects of well-being. This holistic perspective encourages individuals to adopt a well-rounded approach, considering the impact of emotions on their overall quality of life.

Emotional health is a crucial dimension of the holistic approach to well-being, focusing on understanding, expressing, and effectively managing emotions. It encourages individuals to develop emotional intelligence, use healthy coping mechanisms, and recognize the interconnectedness of emotional health with mental and physical well-being. By nurturing emotional health, individuals can enhance their resilience, improve relationships, and experience a greater sense of overall well-being.

Social Health:

Social health is a pivotal dimension of the holistic approach to well-being, focusing on our relationships and interactions with others. It underscores the importance of cultivating and maintaining healthy social connections, fostering positive relationships, and building a supportive social network. Recognizing and nurturing social health is essential for achieving a fulfilling and balanced life.

Healthy Social Connections, Social health begins with establishing and maintaining healthy connections with others. These connections can include family, friends, colleagues, and community members. Healthy relationships are characterized by mutual respect, trust, and open communication. They provide a sense of belonging and support, contributing to emotional well-being.

Positive Relationships, in addition to healthy connections, social health places a strong emphasis on fostering positive relationships. Positive relationships are those that bring joy, fulfillment, and a sense of shared purpose. These relationships are marked by empathy, kindness, and the ability to navigate conflicts constructively. They enhance emotional well-being and provide a valuable source of emotional support during challenging times.

Supportive Social Network, A supportive social network is a vital component of social health. This network consists of individuals who can offer emotional, practical, and social support when needed. Having a strong support system can help individuals cope with stress, overcome adversity, and maintain a sense of resilience. It also provides opportunities for personal growth and a sense of connection to a larger community.

Interconnectedness with Overall Well-Being, Social health has a profound impact on an individual's overall well-being. Research has shown that strong social connections are associated with improved mental and physical health outcomes. Conversely, social isolation and loneliness can lead to negative health effects, including increased risk of depression, anxiety, and chronic diseases. Recognizing the influence of social health on other dimensions of well-being is a key aspect of the holistic approach.

A holistic approach to social health involves recognizing the interconnectedness of social well-being with other aspects of life. It acknowledges that social health influences mental, emotional, physical, and even spiritual well-being. Thus, individuals are encouraged to consider their social connections and relationships as integral components of their overall wellness plan.

Spiritual Health:

Spiritual health is a deeply personal and subjective dimension of the holistic approach to well-being. It involves the search for meaning and purpose in life, connecting with one's inner self, and exploring one's beliefs and values. While spirituality can encompass religious practices for some, it goes beyond organized religion and often involves a quest for a deeper sense of purpose and connection to the universe.

Finding Meaning and Purpose, Spiritual health involves seeking and finding meaning and purpose in life. This quest often revolves around existential questions, such as the purpose of one's existence, the nature of the self, and the significance of human experiences. Finding answers to these questions can provide a sense of fulfillment and contentment.

Inner self-exploration is a central aspect of spiritual health. It encourages individuals to delve into their innermost thoughts, feelings, and beliefs. Practices like meditation, mindfulness, journaling, and self-reflection are commonly used to connect with the inner self and gain deeper insights into one's values and aspirations.

Beliefs and Values, Spiritual health encompasses exploring one's beliefs and values, which may include religious or philosophical beliefs. It's a deeply personal journey that allows individuals to align their actions and choices with their core values. This alignment can lead to a sense of authenticity and inner peace.

Connection to Something Greater, many people seek spiritual health by cultivating a sense of connection to something greater than themselves, whether that's a higher power, the universe, nature, or a collective human consciousness. This connection can provide comfort, guidance, and a sense of belonging.

Holistic Approach to Spiritual Health, A holistic approach to spiritual health acknowledges that spirituality is unique to everyone. It encourages individuals to explore and nurture their spiritual well-being in a way that resonates with them personally. This may involve religious practices, nature-based spirituality, or simply finding moments of stillness and reflection in daily life.

The Interconnectedness of Mind, Body, and Spirit

Central to the holistic approach is the recognition of the intricate interplay between the mind, body, and spirit. These three facets of our existence are not isolated but are deeply intertwined, and disturbances in one area can affect the others. Let's explore this interconnectedness:

1. **Mind-Body Connection:** The mind and body are in constant communication. Psychological stress, for example, can lead to physical symptoms like headaches or digestive issues. Similarly, physical ailments can impact mental health, causing anxiety or depression. Practices like yoga and meditation exemplify how nurturing the mind can positively influence the body's well-being.

2. **Body-Spirit Connection:** Our physical health can also be closely tied to our spiritual well-being. Many traditional healing systems recognize the role of the spirit or inner self in maintaining physical health. Practices like Tai Chi and Qi Gong emphasize the connection between physical movements and spiritual harmony.

3. **Mind-Spirit Connection:** Our mental and emotional states can profoundly impact our spiritual well-being. For instance, cultivating a calm and focused mind through meditation can deepen one's spiritual experiences. Conversely, unresolved emotional issues may hinder spiritual growth and connection.

Understanding these interconnections is essential for achieving holistic well-being. When one aspect of our health is neglected or imbalanced, it can have ripple effects throughout our entire being. Therefore, the holistic approach encourages a comprehensive and integrated approach to health care.

Intermittent Fasting as a Tool for Holistic Well-Being

Intermittent fasting (IF) is a dietary approach that has gained significant attention in recent years as a tool for improving holistic well-being. IF involves cycling between periods of eating and fasting, with various methods and schedules available. Let's explore how IF fits into the holistic approach.

1. **Physical Health:** IF has been associated with several physical health benefits. During fasting periods, the body goes through processes like autophagy, which involves the removal of damaged cells and cellular components. This can contribute to improved cellular health and longevity. Additionally, IF can help with weight management, blood sugar control, and reducing the risk of chronic diseases.

2. **Mental Health:** Fasting can also have effects on mental health. Some people report increased mental clarity and focus during fasting periods. However, it's essential to approach fasting

with mindfulness and ensure it doesn't lead to unhealthy eating behaviors or trigger anxiety.

3. **Emotional Health:** IF may influence emotional health through its impact on hormones and neurotransmitters. For some individuals, stabilizing blood sugar levels through IF can lead to more stable moods. However, it's crucial to be aware of potential emotional challenges that may arise during fasting and address them appropriately.

4. **Spiritual Health:** Intermittent fasting has been practiced in various religious and spiritual traditions as a means of purification and spiritual growth. Fasting can create a sense of discipline and focus, facilitating a deeper connection with one's spiritual beliefs and practices.

It's important to note that while IF can offer potential benefits, it may not be suitable for everyone. Individuals with certain medical conditions or those who are pregnant, or breastfeeding should consult with a healthcare provider before starting any fasting regimen.

The holistic approach to well-being recognizes that well-being encompasses physical, mental, emotional, social, and spiritual dimensions. It emphasizes the interconnectedness of mind, body, and spirit and encourages a comprehensive approach to health care. Intermittent fasting is one dietary strategy that aligns with this approach by potentially benefiting multiple dimensions of well-being. However, it's essential to approach IF with awareness and consideration of individual health needs and goals.

Chapter 2:

Understanding Intermittent Fasting

In recent years, intermittent fasting (IF) has gained widespread attention as a dietary strategy that not only promotes weight loss but also offers potential health benefits for various aspects of well-being. In this chapter, we will delve into the concept of intermittent fasting, explaining what it is, its potential benefits, different fasting protocols, and the scientific rationale behind this fasting approach.

What Is Intermittent Fasting?

Intermittent fasting (IF) is an eating pattern that cycles between periods of fasting and eating. Unlike traditional diets that focus on specific foods or calorie restrictions, IF is more concerned with when you eat rather than what you eat. It doesn't dictate the types of foods to consume but rather the timing of your meals.

The fundamental principle of intermittent fasting is to create extended periods of time where you abstain from food, allowing your body to utilize stored energy and promote various physiological changes. The duration of fasting and eating windows can vary depending on the specific fasting protocol you choose to follow.

Potential Benefits of Intermittent Fasting

Intermittent fasting has garnered attention for its potential health benefits, which extend beyond weight management. While individual results may vary, here are some of the potential advantages associated with intermittent fasting:

Weight Loss:

One of the most widely recognized and celebrated benefits of intermittent fasting is its effectiveness in promoting weight loss. The mechanism behind this weight loss is straightforward: by imposing time-restricted eating windows, individuals naturally reduce their calorie intake. When the body consistently receives fewer calories than it expends, it enters a state of caloric deficit, which, over time, leads to weight loss.

Additionally, intermittent fasting may have a dual effect on weight management:

- **Enhanced Fat Oxidation**: During fasting periods, when glucose stores are depleted, the body shifts to using stored fat as its primary energy source. This process, known as fat oxidation, contributes to the reduction of fat mass.

- **Increased Metabolic** Rate: Some studies suggest that intermittent fasting may boost metabolic rate, particularly during fasting periods. A heightened metabolic rate means the body expends more energy, further supporting weight loss efforts.

It's important to note that while intermittent fasting can be an effective tool for weight management, it should be practiced responsibly and in a way that aligns with individual health goals and needs.

Improved Insulin Sensitivity:

Intermittent fasting can lead to significant improvements in insulin sensitivity, a crucial factor in regulating blood sugar levels. Insulin is a hormone responsible for helping cells absorb glucose (sugar) from the bloodstream. Insulin resistance, where cells become less responsive to insulin's signal, can lead to elevated blood sugar levels and, ultimately, type 2 diabetes.

Intermittent fasting can help enhance insulin sensitivity by:

- **Reducing Meal Frequency:** Fewer meals during the fasting window means fewer spikes in blood sugar levels throughout the day, reducing the strain on the insulin-producing cells in the pancreas.

- **Encouraging Glucose** Regulation: Fasting periods give the body an opportunity to effectively regulate glucose levels, reducing the risk of insulin resistance and promoting stable blood sugar.

For individuals with prediabetes or type 2 diabetes, intermittent fasting may be an effective complementary approach to managing blood sugar levels. However, it's essential to consult with a healthcare provider before making any significant dietary changes, especially if you have a preexisting medical condition.

Cellular Autophagy:

Intermittent fasting triggers a process called autophagy, which translates to "self-eating." This cellular mechanism is a natural housekeeping process that allows the body to identify and remove damaged or dysfunctional cells and cellular components. Think of it as a form of cellular recycling.

Autophagy serves several critical functions:

- **Cellular Cleansing**: By clearing out damaged cellular components, autophagy helps maintain cellular health and functionality.

- **Longevity and Anti-Aging:** The removal of damaged cells is believed to contribute to longevity and may play a role in delaying the aging process.

- **Disease Prevention:** Autophagy may help protect against various diseases, including neurodegenerative disorders, by clearing away misfolded proteins that contribute to disease progression.

Intermittent fasting, particularly during extended fasting periods, is a potent stimulator of autophagy. This cellular cleansing process is often cited as a key factor in the potential health benefits associated with fasting.

Heart Health:

Some evidence suggests that intermittent fasting may lead to improvements in cardiovascular health by addressing risk factors associated with heart disease:

- **Blood Pressure:** Intermittent fasting may help lower blood pressure, reducing the risk of hypertension, a significant risk factor for heart disease.

- **Cholesterol Levels:** Fasting has been linked to favorable changes in cholesterol profiles, including reductions in LDL ("bad") cholesterol and triglycerides.

- **Inflammation:** Chronic inflammation plays a role in the development of cardiovascular disease. Intermittent fasting may help reduce markers of inflammation in the body.

While these findings are promising, it's essential to emphasize that intermittent fasting should not replace other established strategies for heart health, such as a balanced diet and regular physical activity. Instead, it can be integrated into an overall heart-healthy lifestyle.

Brain Health:

Fasting has been associated with potential benefits for brain health and cognitive function:

- **Brain-Derived Neurotrophic Factor (BDNF):** Intermittent fasting may increase the production of BDNF, a protein essential for promoting the growth and maintenance of neurons. Higher BDNF levels are linked to improved cognitive function, memory, and learning.

- **Mental Clarity:** Many individuals report heightened mental clarity and focus during fasting periods, which can be attributed to increased BDNF production and a reduction in blood sugar fluctuations.

- **Neuroprotection:** Fasting may offer neuroprotection by reducing oxidative stress and inflammation in the brain, which are factors in neurodegenerative diseases like Alzheimer's and Parkinson's.

It's important to note that while there is promising research on the potential cognitive benefits of intermittent fasting, more extensive human studies are needed to fully understand its long-term impact on brain health.

Longevity:

Research conducted on animals, particularly rodents, has suggested that intermittent fasting may extend lifespan and promote longevity. These studies have shown that fasting can induce various mechanisms associated with increased longevity, such as improved insulin sensitivity, reduced inflammation, and enhanced cellular repair processes.

However, it's important to approach claims of increased human longevity with caution. While animal studies provide valuable insights, human biology is complex, and more research is needed to establish a definitive link between intermittent fasting and extended lifespan in humans.

Cancer Prevention:

Some animal studies have indicated that intermittent fasting may help protect against cancer by inhibiting the growth of tumors. Fasting may create an environment in which cancer cells struggle to thrive while promoting the body's natural defense mechanisms against cancer development.

It's crucial to emphasize that while these findings are intriguing, they are based on animal studies, and the translation of these effects to humans is not yet fully understood. Cancer is a complex disease, and its prevention and treatment require a multifaceted approach that goes beyond diet alone.

Intermittent fasting offers a range of potential health benefits beyond weight management. These advantages include improved insulin sensitivity, cellular autophagy, heart health, brain health, longevity, and potential cancer prevention. While the scientific evidence supporting these benefits is growing, it's essential to approach intermittent fasting with careful consideration of individual health needs and to consult with healthcare professionals before making significant dietary changes. Researchers continue to explore the full extent of intermittent fasting's impact on human health, and ongoing studies may provide further insights into its long-term effects.

Different Fasting Protocols

Intermittent fasting offers flexibility, allowing individuals to choose from various fasting protocols based on their preferences and lifestyle. Here are some of the most common fasting methods:

16:8 Method:

The 16:8 method is one of the most popular and user-friendly intermittent fasting approaches. It involves fasting for 16 hours each day and restricting eating to an 8-hour window. Here's how it works:

Fasting Period: During the fasting period, which typically begins after dinner and extends through the night, you abstain from consuming any calories. You may drink water, herbal tea, or black coffee, but no solid foods are consumed.

Eating Window: The 8-hour eating window occurs during the daytime. For example, if you start eating at 12:00 PM, you will finish your last meal or snack by 8:00 PM.

The 16:8 method is flexible and can be adjusted to fit your daily routine. Many individuals find it relatively easy to adopt since it allows them to skip breakfast and eat their first meal at lunchtime.

5:2 Method:

The 5:2 method, also known as the "Fast Diet," involves regular eating for five days of the week and restricting calorie intake on the remaining two non-consecutive days. Here's how it typically works:

Regular Eating Days: On the five regular eating days, you consume your usual diet without specific restrictions.

Fasting Days: On the two fasting days, you significantly reduce calorie intake to around 500-600 calories. This can be achieved by consuming low-calorie foods or a small, balanced meal. Fasting days should not be consecutive.

The 5:2 method offers flexibility and allows individuals to maintain a relatively normal eating routine most of the week while experiencing intermittent fasting's benefits on fasting days.

Alternate-Day Fasting:

As the name suggests, alternate day fasting involves alternating between days of fasting and non-fasting. This method offers a variety of approaches:

Full Fasting Days: On fasting days, calorie intake is minimal or eliminated entirely. Some individuals choose to consume only water or non-caloric beverages on these days.

Modified Fasting Days: Others opt for a modified approach, where they consume a limited number of calories, typically around 500-600 calories, on fasting days.

Alternate day fasting can be challenging for some people due to the alternating nature of the regimen. However, it may be effective for those looking for a more intensive intermittent fasting experience.

OMAD (One Meal a Day):

OMAD, or One Meal a Day, is a straightforward and restrictive fasting protocol. In this approach:

Eating Window: You consume all your daily calories within a single one-hour to two-hour eating window. The rest of the day is spent fasting.

Fasting Duration: Fasting can last from 22 to 23 hours, depending on the duration of your chosen eating window.

OMAD requires a significant amount of discipline and can be challenging for those who are accustomed to regular meals throughout the day. It may not be suitable for everyone, especially those with specific dietary needs or health conditions.

Eat-Stop-Eat:

Eat-Stop-Eat is an intermittent fasting method that involves fasting for a full 24 hours once or twice a week. Here's how it works:

Fasting Period: You abstain from food and calorie-containing beverages for a 24-hour period. For instance, if you finish dinner at 7:00 PM, you will not eat again until 7:00 PM the following day.

Non-Fasting Days: On non-fasting days, you maintain your regular eating pattern.

Eat-Stop-Eat offers a break from regular eating without requiring daily fasting. It provides flexibility by allowing you to choose fasting days that align with your schedule and preferences.

Warrior Diet:

The Warrior Diet is a fasting method that combines an extended fasting period with a shorter eating window. Here's how it typically works:

Fasting Period: You fast for 20 hours each day, during which you consume only minimal calories from raw fruits and vegetables or small snacks.

Eating Window: The eating window spans a 4-hour period, usually in the evening. This is when the main meal of the day is consumed.

The Warrior Diet is named for its association with ancient warriors who consumed one large meal after returning from battle. It can be challenging due to the extended fasting period but allows for a substantial meal in the evening.

Extended Fasting:

Extended fasting refers to fasting periods that extend beyond 48 hours, often lasting several days or up to a week. Extended fasts should be undertaken with caution and preferably under medical supervision.

Extended fasting can offer more profound benefits such as enhanced autophagy and a reset of metabolic processes. However, it requires careful planning, hydration, and attention to electrolyte balance to ensure safety.

Scientific Rationale Behind Intermittent Fasting

The scientific rationale behind intermittent fasting lies in its ability to induce various physiological changes that can promote health and well-being.

Caloric Restriction:

Intermittent fasting's effectiveness in promoting health and well-being is rooted in its ability to impose a form of caloric restriction. Caloric restriction involves reducing calorie intake without malnutrition, and it has been extensively studied for its potential health benefits. Intermittent fasting achieves this caloric reduction by limiting the time available for eating. Here's how it works:

Calorie Deficit: By reducing the number of hours available for eating, intermittent fasting naturally restricts calorie intake. This caloric deficit leads to weight loss over time, as the body expends more energy than it receives from food.

Longevity: Caloric restriction has been shown to extend lifespan in various organisms, including yeast, worms, flies, and rodents. While the direct translation to human longevity is not fully established, it suggests a potential link between intermittent fasting and increased lifespan.

Metabolic Health: Caloric restriction improves metabolic health by promoting insulin sensitivity and reducing the risk of metabolic diseases like type 2 diabetes. It also encourages the body to use stored fat for energy, contributing to weight management.

Hormone Regulation:

Intermittent fasting has a profound impact on hormone regulation, leading to various health benefits:

Human Growth Hormone (HGH): Fasting triggers an increase in HGH levels. HGH plays a crucial role in fat metabolism, muscle preservation, and overall growth and repair processes. Elevated HGH levels during fasting can promote fat burning and muscle preservation.

Insulin: Fasting leads to decreased insulin levels. Lower insulin levels reduce the body's storage of glucose as fat, promoting fat breakdown for energy. Improved insulin sensitivity can also reduce the risk of insulin resistance and type 2 diabetes.

Norepinephrine: Fasting stimulates the release of norepinephrine, a hormone and neurotransmitter that increases alertness and enhances fat mobilization. This hormone helps the body utilize stored fat for energy.

Glucagon: Fasting elevates glucagon levels, which promotes the breakdown of stored glycogen into glucose for energy. This process helps maintain stable blood sugar levels during fasting periods.

Autophagy:

Autophagy, meaning "self-eating," is a cellular process stimulated by fasting. It serves as a critical mechanism for cellular repair and maintenance:

Cellular Cleansing: Autophagy involves the removal and recycling of damaged or dysfunctional cellular components, including proteins and organelles. This process keeps cells healthy and functioning optimally.

Longevity: Autophagy has been linked to increased longevity in various organisms. By removing cellular waste and repairing damage, it may help prevent age-related diseases and extend lifespan.

Disease Prevention: Autophagy plays a role in protecting against neurodegenerative diseases, infections, and cancer by eliminating misfolded proteins, damaged organelles, and potentially harmful intracellular invaders.

Inflammation Reduction:

Chronic inflammation is a common denominator in many chronic diseases. Intermittent fasting has been shown to reduce markers of inflammation in the body:

Cytokine Regulation: Fasting helps regulate the production of pro-inflammatory cytokines, which are signaling molecules involved in the inflammatory response. Reducing excessive inflammation can lower the risk of chronic diseases.

Oxidative Stress: Fasting may reduce oxidative stress, which occurs when there's an imbalance between free radicals and antioxidants in the body. Lower oxidative stress is associated with improved health and reduced inflammation.

Brain Health:

Fasting has a significant impact on brain health and cognitive function:

Brain-Derived Neurotrophic Factor (BDNF): Fasting promotes the release of BDNF, a protein crucial for neuronal growth, plasticity, and survival. Higher BDNF levels are associated with improved cognitive function, mood regulation, and overall brain health.

Mental Clarity: Many individuals report heightened mental clarity and focus during fasting periods. This enhanced mental state is attributed to factors like increased BDNF levels and reduced blood sugar fluctuations.

Neuroprotection: Fasting may provide neuroprotection by reducing oxidative stress and inflammation in the brain, factors linked to neurodegenerative diseases such as Alzheimer's and Parkinson's.

Cellular Longevity:

Intermittent fasting has been linked to cellular longevity and the preservation of cellular health:

Oxidative Stress Management: Fasting can reduce oxidative stress in cells, which is a contributing factor to cellular aging and damage. By managing oxidative stress, fasting may help maintain cellular integrity.

DNA Repair: Autophagy processes stimulated by fasting can assist in DNA repair and maintenance, reducing the risk of mutations and cellular dysfunction.

Metabolic Flexibility:

Fasting encourages the body to shift from using glucose as its primary fuel source to burning stored fat for energy. This metabolic flexibility offers several benefits:

Weight Management: Metabolic flexibility allows for effective fat burning, aiding in weight management and reducing the risk of obesity-related conditions.

Energy Balance: Fasting helps regulate energy balance by allowing the body to tap into stored fat reserves when needed. This ensures a steady supply of energy even during fasting periods.

Intermittent fasting offers a compelling scientific rationale for its potential health benefits. It leverages mechanisms such as caloric restriction, hormone regulation, autophagy, inflammation reduction, brain health promotion, cellular longevity, and metabolic flexibility to support overall well-being. However, it's crucial to approach intermittent fasting mindfully and consider individual health needs. Consulting with a healthcare professional before starting any fasting regimen is advisable, particularly for those with underlying medical conditions or unique dietary requirements. Part II of this book will provide practical guidance on incorporating intermittent fasting into a holistic approach to health and well-being.

Chapter 3:

Mindful Living and Mindfulness Practices

As we begin on this holistic journey, it is essential to recognize the vital role of mindfulness in achieving well-being that encompasses the mind, body, and spirit. In this chapter, we will explore the importance of mindful living and introduce mindfulness practices that can enrich your life.

The Importance of Mindfulness in Holistic Health

In the quest for holistic health and well-being, the role of mindfulness cannot be overstated. Mindfulness is not just a trendy concept; it is a profound way of life that can deeply influence and transform every facet of your being. At its essence, mindfulness entails being fully present in the moment, without judgment or distraction. It involves cultivating an acute awareness of your thoughts, emotions, and physical sensations, as well as the world that surrounds you.

The Modern Challenge

In today's fast-paced, hyperconnected world, we often find ourselves engulfed in a whirlwind of distractions. The constant barrage of information, digital devices, and hectic schedules can make it challenging to stay grounded and truly connected to our own inner selves and the world around us. This lack of connection and presence can take a toll on our holistic well-being, impacting not only our mental and emotional states but also our physical health.

The Mindfulness Solution

Mindfulness provides a powerful antidote to the modern-day challenges we face. By actively engaging in mindfulness practices, we can reintroduce a sense of balance and harmony into our lives. Here's why mindfulness is so vital in the context of holistic health:

Stress Reduction: Mindfulness serves as a potent tool for managing and reducing stress. In the practice of mindfulness, you learn to observe your thoughts and emotions without judgment. This nonjudgmental awareness can help you disengage from the cycle of stress, allowing you to respond to challenging situations with greater calm and resilience.

Emotional Regulation: Mindfulness empowers you to develop a more profound understanding of your emotional landscape. It enables you to acknowledge and accept your emotions without becoming overwhelmed by them. By doing so, you can navigate emotional turbulence with grace and make healthier choices in how you respond to your feelings.

Enhanced Well-Being: Engaging in mindfulness practices can lead to a profound sense of well-being. As you become more present in your daily life, you start to appreciate the beauty in the simplest of moments—a vibrant sunset, the warmth of a smile, or the taste of a nourishing meal. These moments of presence and appreciation add depth and richness to your overall sense of well-being.

Improved Physical Health: Mindfulness isn't confined to the realm of the mind and emotions; it has tangible effects on physical health. Research has shown that mindfulness practices can reduce blood pressure, improve sleep quality, boost immune function, and even alleviate chronic pain. This mind-body connection underscores the holistic nature of mindfulness.

Enhanced Relationships: Mindfulness also extends its benefits to our interactions with others. When you practice mindfulness, you become a better listener, more empathetic, and less reactive in your relationships. This can lead to more profound and fulfilling connections with friends, family, and colleagues.

Cultivation of Gratitude: Mindfulness encourages the cultivation of gratitude. By paying attention to the present moment and acknowledging the positive aspects of your life, you can foster a sense of appreciation and contentment. Gratitude is a powerful force that can enhance your overall well-being.

Self-Awareness and Growth: Mindfulness is a journey of self-discovery and personal growth. It encourages you to explore the depths of your own mind and heart, uncovering hidden beliefs, patterns, and potentials. This self-awareness can be a catalyst for positive change and personal evolution.

Introducing Mindfulness Techniques

In this section, we will introduce you to a variety of mindfulness techniques that can seamlessly integrate into your daily life. These practices are designed to help you cultivate mindfulness, which is the art of being fully present in the moment and developing an awareness of your thoughts, emotions, and bodily sensations without judgment. By incorporating these techniques into your routine, you can promote inner peace, reduce stress, and enhance your overall well-being.

Meditation:

Meditation stands as a cornerstone of mindfulness practice. It encompasses various techniques and approaches that guide you towards a state of heightened awareness and tranquility. Here are some types of meditation you can explore:

Mindfulness Meditation: This form of meditation involves paying attention to your breath, bodily sensations, and thoughts as they arise without judgment. It's an excellent practice for grounding yourself in the present moment.

Loving-Kindness Meditation: Loving-kindness meditation focuses on cultivating feelings of compassion and love, both for yourself and others. It involves repeating phrases or affirmations that promote goodwill and empathy.

Body Scan Meditation: In body scan meditation, you systematically scan your body from head to toe, directing your attention to each part. This practice enhances your awareness of bodily sensations and promotes relaxation.

Meditation doesn't require a significant time commitment. Even just a few minutes of daily practice can yield noticeable benefits, such as reduced stress and improved focus. Over time, you can tailor your meditation routine to suit your preferences and needs.

Deep Breathing:

Deep breathing is a simple yet potent mindfulness tool that you can utilize anytime and anywhere. It involves conscious, deliberate breath control to anchor yourself in the present moment. Here's how to incorporate deep breathing into your daily life:

Breath Awareness: Start by bringing your attention to your breath. Notice the sensation of the breath entering and leaving your body. You can place your hand on your abdomen to feel the rise and fall as you breathe.

Slow, Deep Breaths: Take slow, deep breaths, inhaling deeply through your nose and exhaling slowly through your mouth. Count to four as you inhale, hold for a moment, and then count to four as you exhale. Repeat this cycle several times.

Focused Breathing: You can also combine deep breathing with a simple focus point, such as a calming word or phrase. Inhale as you silently say, "I am," and exhale as you say, "at peace." This helps synchronize your breath with positive affirmations.

Deep breathing can be particularly effective in reducing stress and anxiety. It provides a quick way to center yourself and regain a sense of calm during challenging moments.

Mindful Eating:

Eating can be a profoundly mindful experience when approached with awareness and intention. Mindful eating encourages you to savor each bite, fully appreciating the flavors, textures, and sensations of your food. Here's how to practice mindful eating:

Eliminate Distractions: When you eat, create a calm and focused environment. Turn off screens, put away your phone, and sit down at a designated eating space.

Engage Your Senses: Before taking a bite, take a moment to observe your food. Notice its colors, shapes, and textures. Inhale the aroma and appreciate the presentation.

Eat Slowly: Take your time with each bite. Chew slowly and deliberately, savoring the flavors. Put your utensils down between bites to fully experience the meal.

Be Present: Pay attention to how your body responds to each bite. Notice the sensations of hunger and fullness. Tune in to any emotional or psychological responses to the food.

Practicing mindful eating not only enhances your enjoyment of meals but can also support healthier eating habits. By being present during meals, you can better recognize hunger cues and make mindful choices about what and how much you eat.

Practical Tips for Embracing Mindfulness

The beauty of mindfulness lies in its simplicity and accessibility. You don't need any special equipment or lengthy time commitments to experience its transformative effects. Mindfulness can be seamlessly integrated into your daily life, enriching your overall well-being. In this chapter, we'll provide you with practical tips to help you effortlessly incorporate mindfulness into your daily routine.

Morning Rituals:

Starting your day with a mindful morning routine can set a positive tone for the hours ahead. Here's how to infuse mindfulness into your mornings:

Wake Up Mindfully: Begin by waking up with intention. Take a few moments to stretch and breathe deeply. Express gratitude for the new day and the opportunities it brings.

Mindful Breathing: Incorporate deep breathing exercises into your morning routine. As you wash your face or brush your teeth, focus on your breath to ground yourself in the present moment.

Mindful Breakfast: When you have breakfast, eat mindfully. Savor each bite, paying attention to the taste, texture, and aroma of your food. Avoid rushing through your meal.

Set Intentions: Take a moment to set positive intentions for the day. Consider what you hope to achieve and how you want to show up in various aspects of your life.

A mindful morning routine can enhance your sense of purpose and create a peaceful foundation for the day ahead.

Mindful Walking:

Walking mindfully is a practice that can be enjoyed anywhere, whether in a serene natural setting or amidst the hustle and bustle of a busy city. Here's how to incorporate mindful walking into your daily life:

Choose Your Path: Find a location where you can walk safely and comfortably. This could be a park, a nature trail, or even a quiet street in your neighborhood.

Walk Slowly: As you walk, slow down your pace. Pay attention to each step and the sensations of your feet touching the ground.

Engage Your Senses: Use all your senses to immerse yourself in the experience. Notice the sounds around you, the colors of nature, and the feel of the air on your skin.

Breathe Mindfully: Sync your breath with your steps. Inhale as you take a step, and exhale as you take the next. This rhythmic breathing can help you stay present.

Mindful walking allows you to connect with the world around you and can be a calming and grounding practice.

Technology Detox:

In our digitally connected world, it's essential to unplug from devices and create moments of digital-free mindfulness. Here's how to incorporate technology detox into your daily life:

Designate Tech-Free Zones: Identify areas in your home where technology is not allowed, such as the bedroom or the dining table. This promotes more meaningful connections with loved ones.

Set Boundaries: Establish specific times of day when you disconnect from screens. Use this time to engage in mindfulness practices or simply enjoy real-world experiences.

Mindful Tech Use: When you do use technology, do so mindfully. Be conscious of how much time you spend on screens and how it makes you feel. Consider apps or tools that help limit screen time.

Nature Retreat: Spend time in nature without the distraction of technology. Take a hike, have a picnic, or simply sit under a tree and observe the natural world around you.

A technology detox allows you to reconnect with yourself, your surroundings, and the people in your life.

Mindful Relationships:

Mindfulness can significantly enhance your relationships by fostering better communication, empathy, and connection. Here's how to incorporate mindfulness into your interactions with others:

Active Listening: When engaging in conversations, practice active listening. Give the speaker your full attention, without interrupting or formulating your response prematurely.

Empathy and Understanding: Try to see the world from the perspective of the other person. Cultivate empathy by acknowledging their feelings and experiences.

Pause Before Reacting: Instead of reacting impulsively in challenging situations, take a mindful pause. Breathe deeply and consider your response carefully.

Gratitude in Relationships: Express gratitude for the people in your life. Let them know how much you appreciate their presence and support.

Mindful relationships are built on empathy, respect, and authentic connections, leading to more harmonious and fulfilling interactions.

Understand the profound impact of mindfulness on your holistic well-being but also have practical tools at your disposal to start living a more mindful and enriching life. Mindfulness is the thread that weaves through the tapestry of holistic health, connecting the mind, body, and spirit in a beautiful symphony of self-awareness and growth. With these practical tips, you can embrace mindfulness as an integral part of your daily life, nurturing your overall well-being and fostering a deeper sense of presence and connection with the world around you.

Chapter 4:
Nourishing the Spirit

In the pursuit of holistic well-being, it's essential to recognize that health goes beyond the physical and mental realms. The spiritual dimension plays a profound and integral role in our overall sense of well-being. In this chapter, we will delve into the spiritual dimension of well-being, exploring practices and concepts that can nourish the spirit and enhance our holistic health. We'll discuss the importance of spirituality, various spiritual practices such as gratitude and journaling, and how nurturing the spirit can contribute to overall health.

The Spiritual Dimension of Well-Being

The spiritual dimension of well-being encompasses our sense of purpose, connection to something greater than ourselves, and our innermost beliefs and values. It transcends religious affiliation and dogma, as it is a deeply personal and subjective aspect of our existence. Here are some key elements of the spiritual dimension:

Meaning and Purpose:

At the heart of spirituality lies the quest for meaning and purpose in life. It is a journey of self-discovery that involves profound questions about our existence, our role in the world, and what imbues our lives with significance. This search for meaning serves as a guiding force, leading us to explore our passions, values, and what truly matters to us. It propels us to seek out experiences and connections that align with our innermost desires and aspirations.

Connection:

Spirituality often entails a sense of profound connection or oneness with the universe, nature, or a higher power. It extends beyond the boundaries of the self and fosters a deep feeling of interconnectedness with all living beings.

This connection can manifest in various ways, from a reverence for the natural world to a sense of unity with the collective human experience. It reminds us that we are not isolated entities but integral parts of a vast, interconnected web of life.

Values and Beliefs:

Our spiritual dimension is profoundly shaped by our values and beliefs. These values serve as guiding principles that inform our decisions, actions, and ethical conduct. They provide us with a moral compass that steers us toward what we perceive as right and just. Spirituality encourages us to reflect on our values and beliefs, fostering a deeper understanding of our ethical foundations and influencing our interactions with the world and others.

Transcendence:

Spirituality often leads to experiences of transcendence, where individuals transcend their everyday consciousness and glimpse something greater or divine. These moments can be deeply transformative, evoking feelings of awe, wonder, and reverence. Whether through meditation, prayer, or encounters with the natural world, these experiences offer a glimpse beyond the boundaries of the material world, igniting a sense of profound connection to the cosmos.

Moral and Ethical Development:

Many spiritual traditions emphasize the importance of moral and ethical development. They encourage individuals to cultivate virtues such as compassion, kindness, forgiveness, and empathy. These values serve not only as ethical guidelines but also as pathways to personal growth and inner peace. By nurturing these virtues, individuals can foster more harmonious relationships, contribute positively to their communities, and live in alignment with their spiritual beliefs.

The spiritual dimension of well-being is a multifaceted and deeply personal aspect of our existence. It invites us to explore the depths of our inner selves, seek meaning and purpose, and cultivate values that guide our actions and decisions. It encourages us to connect with something greater than ourselves, whether through experiences of transcendence or a profound sense of interconnectedness with all living beings. Ultimately, the spiritual dimension reminds us that our journey toward holistic well-being encompasses not only physical and mental health but also a profound exploration of our inner worlds and our place in the grand tapestry of existence.

Practices to Nourish the Spirit

Nourishing the spirit is an essential part of holistic well-being, as it fosters a sense of purpose, connection, and inner growth. Engaging in spiritual practices can help individuals explore the depths of their inner selves and cultivate a profound sense of fulfillment. Here are some practices that can nurture the spiritual dimension of well-being:

Gratitude:

Cultivating gratitude is a powerful spiritual practice that has the potential to transform our outlook on life. It involves acknowledging and appreciating the blessings, both big and small, that grace our lives. By intentionally focusing on gratitude, we shift our perspective from what we lack to what we have, fostering contentment and a profound sense of abundance. This practice encourages us to recognize the beauty and richness in everyday moments, from the warmth of a sunrise to the kindness of a stranger.

Journaling:

Keeping a journal serves as a means of self-reflection and spiritual exploration. Through the act of journaling, we start on a journey of self-discovery, diving into the depths of our thoughts, feelings, and experiences. It provides a sacred space for us to express our innermost thoughts and emotions, gain insights into our inner world, and track our personal growth over time. Journaling can serve as a powerful tool for self-awareness, allowing us to explore our beliefs, values, and aspirations.

Meditation:

Meditation is a versatile and profound practice that has the potential to deeply nourish the spirit. It offers a gateway to connect with our inner selves, explore the landscape of our thoughts and emotions, and experience moments of transcendence and clarity. Through meditation, we can cultivate a deep sense of presence and mindfulness, allowing us to become fully aware of each moment as it unfolds. Whether through focused breath awareness, loving-kindness meditation, or body scan meditation, this practice enables us to tap into our inner wisdom and connect with the profound stillness within.

Mindfulness:

As discussed in previous chapters, mindfulness is another practice that nurtures the spirit. It involves the art of being fully present in the moment, without judgment or distraction. Mindfulness invites us to embrace each moment with openness and curiosity, fostering a deeper sense of connection and inner peace. Through mindful awareness, we learn to appreciate the beauty of life's simple pleasures and find solace in the present moment, free from the burdens of the past or anxieties about the future.

Nature Connection:

Spending time in nature is a deeply spiritual practice that can evoke a profound sense of awe, wonder, and interconnectedness. Nature serves as a source of inspiration and reflection, inviting us to step outside the confines of our daily lives and connect with the natural world. Whether it's a walk in the woods, a hike in the mountains, or simply sitting by a tranquil stream, nature offers a sanctuary for introspection and rejuvenation. Through this practice, we can develop a deeper appreciation for the intricate web of life that surrounds us and cultivate a sense of harmony with the Earth.

Acts of Kindness:

Engaging in acts of kindness and service to others is a practice deeply rooted in spirituality. It allows us to connect with our inherent compassion and empathy, fostering a profound sense of purpose and fulfillment. Acts of kindness can range from simple gestures of goodwill, such as helping a neighbor, to more significant acts of service, like volunteering for a charitable organization. By extending kindness to others, we not only contribute positively to their lives but also experience a deep sense of interconnectedness and belonging within our communities.

Finding Purpose:

Exploring and discovering one's purpose in life is a central aspect of the spiritual dimension. It involves a journey of aligning our actions with our deepest values and beliefs, contributing to a meaningful and fulfilling life. Finding purpose can be an ongoing process, as it requires self-reflection, exploration of our passions, and an understanding of how we can make a positive impact on the world. By living in alignment with our purpose, we cultivate a sense of fulfillment that transcends material gains and contributes to our spiritual growth.

How Spirituality Enhances Overall Health

Nurturing the spirit isn't solely about finding inner peace and well-being; it also has a profound impact on our physical and mental health. Here's a closer look at how spirituality enhances health across various dimensions.

Stress Reduction:

Spiritual practices such as meditation and mindfulness can effectively reduce stress by promoting relaxation and emotional regulation. When individuals engage in these practices, they create a sacred space for tranquility and inner peace. By focusing on the present moment, spiritual practices help alleviate anxiety and tension. Furthermore, individuals with a strong sense of purpose and connection often possess better resilience, which can buffer against the negative effects of stress.

Improved Mental Health:

Spirituality is closely associated with better mental health outcomes. Research suggests that individuals who embrace spiritual practices report reduced symptoms of anxiety and depression. Practices such as gratitude and journaling can significantly contribute to emotional well-being. Gratitude encourages a positive outlook, helping individuals reframe their thoughts to focus on the positive aspects of life. Journaling, on the other hand, provides an outlet for expressing emotions and self-reflection, ultimately fostering emotional clarity and resilience.

Enhanced Resilience:

A robust spiritual foundation often serves as a source of strength and resilience during challenging times. It provides individuals with a profound sense of meaning, purpose, and hope, which can be particularly crucial during adversity. Those who have a strong connection to their spirituality tend to exhibit a greater ability to cope with life's difficulties, bounce back from setbacks, and maintain a positive outlook.

Better Physical Health:

Emerging studies suggest that spirituality may have positive effects on physical health. Individuals who engage in spiritual practices may experience lower blood pressure, improved immune function, and a reduced risk of chronic diseases. While the precise mechanisms behind these effects are still under investigation, it is clear that spiritual well-being can have a holistic impact on one's health.

Increased Longevity:

Research has indicated that individuals who possess a strong sense of purpose and spiritual connection tend to live longer and enjoy better health outcomes. A profound sense of purpose can drive individuals to take better care of themselves and make healthier lifestyle choices. It can also instill a greater will to overcome challenges and maintain a zest for life, contributing to increased longevity.

Enhanced Coping Mechanisms:

Spiritual practices offer individuals effective coping mechanisms when facing life's difficulties. Whether through meditation, prayer, or acts of kindness, spirituality equips individuals with the tools to navigate stressors and challenges more healthily. These practices provide solace, insight, and inner strength, allowing individuals to respond to adversity with grace and resilience.

The spiritual dimension of well-being is a deeply personal and meaningful aspect of our existence. It encompasses our sense of purpose, connection, values, and beliefs. Nurturing the spirit through practices like gratitude, journaling, meditation, and acts of kindness is not only about achieving inner peace but also about experiencing profound enhancements in our holistic health. Spirituality serves as the unifying thread that weaves through the tapestry of holistic health, connecting the mind, body, and spirit in a beautiful symphony of self-awareness and growth. It reminds us that well-being is not merely the absence of illness but also about leading a purposeful, meaningful, and fulfilling life. By acknowledging and nurturing our spiritual dimension, we can achieve a more profound and holistic sense of well-being.

Chapter 5:
Preparing for Detox

Beginning a journey of holistic detoxification, whether it's a 14-day program or any other duration, requires thoughtful preparation. Preparing your mind and body adequately can significantly enhance the effectiveness of the detox process and your overall well-being throughout the program. In this chapter, we'll delve into the importance of preparation and provide you with a comprehensive checklist to help you get ready both mentally and physically.

Importance of Preparation

Preparation is the cornerstone upon which the success of your detox program rests. It serves as the vital bridge that connects your current state of being with the transformative journey you're about to begin. Whether your detox program spans 14 days or any other duration, here's why meticulous preparation is of paramount importance:

Mental Readiness:

The process of detoxifying the mind, body, and spirit is inherently transformative. It involves a conscious commitment to change, growth, and self-improvement. Mental preparation equips you with the right mindset, enabling you to set clear goals, intentions, and motivations. It empowers you to embrace change, confront obstacles, and stay steadfastly committed throughout the program. By cultivating mental readiness, you fortify your resolve, making it easier to stay on the path of holistic wellness.

Establishing a Routine:

Detox programs often entail significant changes in your daily life, including modifications to your diet, exercise regimen, and daily habits. Effective preparation allows you to transition into these changes gradually and seamlessly. This gradual shift minimizes the chances of feeling overwhelmed or deprived, enhancing your capacity to adapt and thrive. Moreover, it grants you the opportunity to establish a sustainable routine that extends beyond the program's duration, ensuring that the benefits you reap continue to nourish your holistic well-being.

Gathering Supplies:

The specifics of your detox program, whether they involve specific foods, supplements, or equipment, necessitate meticulous planning and preparation. Gathering the necessary supplies in advance is paramount. This ensures that you have everything readily available when you need it, thus eliminating last-minute stress or interruptions to your carefully designed routine. A well-prepared environment facilitates a smoother detoxification process.

Creating a Support System:

The journey of detoxification can be challenging, and there will likely be moments when you seek encouragement, understanding, or guidance. During the preparation phase, you can inform those in your inner circle—friends, family, or a trusted confidant—about your intentions. By sharing your goals and aspirations, you create a network of support that is invaluable. This support system can provide not only emotional reassurance but also practical assistance when necessary, helping you navigate challenges and celebrate victories together.

Reducing Withdrawal Symptoms:

If your detox program entails reducing or eliminating specific substances, such as caffeine, sugar, or processed foods, preparation allows you to mitigate the potential for withdrawal symptoms. Gradual reduction of these substances, initiated during the preparation phase, can significantly reduce the intensity and duration of withdrawal. This gentle approach is kinder to your body and mind, ensuring a more comfortable transition into the detox program.

In essence, preparation is your compass, guiding you as you begin your holistic detox journey. It's the bedrock upon which your commitment to change and well-being is established. By focusing on mental readiness, routine establishment, gathering supplies, creating a support network, and minimizing withdrawal symptoms, you not only pave the way for a successful detox but also set the stage for profound transformation and holistic wellness.

The Detox Preparation Checklist

Now, let's provide you with a comprehensive checklist to guide you through the preparation process for your mind-body-spirit detox program. Proper preparation ensures a smooth and successful journey:

Mental Preparation:

Mentally preparing for a detox requires a mindset of commitment, self-awareness, and perseverance. Start by setting clear, realistic goals and reflecting on the reasons behind your decision to detoxify. Remind yourself of the potential benefits, such as improved energy levels, better digestion, and enhanced mental clarity. Acknowledge that there may be moments of discomfort or cravings, but also recognize that these are temporary hurdles in your journey towards a healthier lifestyle. Building a strong support system and integrating stress-relief techniques can be invaluable tools in maintaining motivation and navigating through the detox process.

Set Clear Goals

Begin by defining your objectives for the detox program. Are you seeking increased energy, mental clarity, weight loss, emotional well-being, or a combination of these? Knowing your goals will provide a clear sense of purpose and direction throughout the program.

Create a Detox Journal

Consider starting a journal to document your detox journey. In this journal, record your goals, daily experiences, challenges, and successes. Journaling can serve as a valuable tool for self-reflection and tracking your progress.

Establish a Support Network

Share your detox plans with friends or family members. Seek their understanding and, if possible, enlist their support in your journey. Having a support network can offer encouragement and motivation during challenging times.

Mindful Meditation

If you're not already practicing meditation, consider beginning or enhancing your meditation practice. Mindfulness meditation can help you stay present, reduce stress, and enhance self-awareness throughout the program.

Physical Preparation:

Before delving into the process of cleansing and rejuvenating your body, it's crucial to establish a strong foundation by incorporating healthy habits, such as regular exercise, staying hydrated, and maintaining a balanced diet. Engaging in these practices will help your body gradually adapt to the forthcoming changes and ensure a successful detox experience.

Medical Consultation:

Before starting the detox program, consult with a healthcare professional, especially if you have underlying health conditions or are taking medications. Discuss your detox plans with them to ensure they align with your health status.

Gather Supplies

Depending on the specific requirements of your chosen detox program, gather the necessary supplies. This may include fresh produce, herbal teas, supplements, or other detox-friendly items.

Meal Planning

Plan your detox-friendly meals and snacks. Explore recipes that align with your program's guidelines and create a shopping list to ensure you have nutritious options readily available.

Hydration

Start increasing your water intake in the days leading up to the detox program. Proper hydration is crucial for supporting detoxification and overall well-being.

Exercise Routine

If you're not currently engaged in regular physical activity, begin incorporating moderate exercise into your routine. Exercise promotes circulation and sweating, which can aid in the detox process.

Eliminate Stimulants Gradually

If your detox program involves reducing caffeine or sugar intake, start gradually reducing these substances in the days leading up to the program. This gradual reduction can help minimize withdrawal symptoms.

Environmental Preparation:

Preparing for a detox requires creating a serene and uncluttered environment to concentrate and operate effectively. By removing distractions and organizing your space, you can set the stage for a successful cleanse that rejuvenates both mind and body. A clean and organized area facilitates focus, making it easier for you to commit to your detox journey and attain optimal results.

Declutter Your Space

Create a clean and organized environment in your home. A clutter-free space can contribute to a sense of calm and focus during your detox journey.

Create a Peaceful Retreat

Designate a tranquil space within your home where you can practice mindfulness, meditation, or simply relax and unwind. Make this space inviting and conducive to self-care.

Time and Scheduling:

Preparing for a detox requires mindful organization and dedication to achieve the best results. By setting timers and scheduling specific moments to concentrate on your wellbeing, you can effectively create a structured plan to cleanse your body and mind. This intentionality ensures that you have allocated enough time to fully commit to the detox process and maximize its benefits.

Set Start and End Dates

Determine the official start and end dates of your detox program. Having a clear timeframe helps you commit to the program and stay on track.

Plan Your Schedule

Consider how the detox program may impact your daily routine. Make any necessary adjustments to accommodate additional self-care practices, such as meditation, exercise, or meal preparation.

By diligently working through this comprehensive checklist, you'll lay a solid foundation for your 14-day mind-body-spirit detox program. Remember that preparation encompasses both the practical aspects and nurturing the right mindset and support system. With thorough preparation, you'll be better equipped to start your journey, maximize the program's benefits, and foster lasting holistic well-being.

Chapter 6:

Day 1-3: The Physical Cleanse

In the journey of holistic well-being, the first three days are critical. This initial phase, known as the "Physical Cleanse," is dedicated to revitalizing your body, ridding it of toxins, and jumpstarting your path to wellness. During these days, you'll nourish your body with cleansing foods, hydrate it with detoxifying liquids, and engage in gentle exercises to kickstart your metabolism. This chapter will guide you through the first phase of your detox program, offering insights into the importance of a physical cleanse, a structured meal plan tailored to these initial days, and a selection of recipes designed to support detoxification and promote weight loss.

The Importance of the Physical Cleanse

Before delving into the specifics of your meal plan and recipes, let's explore why the physical cleanse is a crucial starting point in your holistic detox journey.

Toxin Elimination:

Over time, our bodies accumulate toxins from various sources, including processed foods, environmental pollutants, and stress. These toxins can lead to fatigue, digestive issues, and weight gain. The physical cleanse focuses on flushing out these toxins to restore vitality and balance.

Metabolic Boost:

By adopting a nutrient-rich, whole-food diet during the initial days, you provide your body with essential vitamins, minerals, and antioxidants. This nourishment supports your metabolism, helping your body efficiently convert food into energy and promote weight loss.

Digestive Reset:

Many detox programs emphasize light, easily digestible foods during the physical cleanse phase. This shift in dietary choices gives your digestive system a break, allowing it to reset and function optimally. Improved digestion leads to better nutrient absorption and overall well-being.

Energy Revival:

Ridding your body of toxins and fueling it with wholesome foods can lead to increased energy levels. As your body cleanses and rejuvenates, you'll likely experience enhanced vitality, mental clarity, and a sense of well-being.

Now, let's dive into the practical aspects of your physical cleanse, starting with a structured meal plan for days 1-3.

Structured Meal Plan for Days 1-3

Note: This meal plan is a general guideline and can be adapted to your dietary preferences and any specific detox program you are following. It is important to consult with a healthcare professional or nutritionist before starting any detox program, especially if you have underlying health conditions or dietary restrictions.

Day 1: Cleansing Start

Morning: Start your day with a glass of warm water with lemon to kickstart digestion. Follow with a green smoothie made from spinach, kale, cucumber, and a touch of fresh ginger.

Mid-Morning Snack: Enjoy a serving of sliced cucumber and carrot sticks with a small portion of hummus for a light and hydrating snack.

Lunch: Savor a detox salad with mixed greens, cherry tomatoes, bell peppers, and a homemade vinaigrette dressing. Top with grilled chicken or tofu for protein.

Afternoon Snack: Have a small serving of plain Greek yogurt or a dairy-free alternative with a drizzle of honey and a sprinkle of chia seeds.

Dinner: opt for a light and nourishing soup, such as a vegetable broth with plenty of leafy greens, carrots, and celery. Add a side of quinoa or brown rice for sustenance.

Evening: Wind down with a cup of herbal tea, such as chamomile or peppermint, to aid digestion and promote relaxation.

Day 2: Nutrient Replenishment

Morning: Begin your day with warm water and a splash of apple cider vinegar. Follow with a berry smoothie made with mixed berries, spinach, and a scoop of plant-based protein powder.

Mid-Morning Snack: Enjoy a handful of mixed nuts and seeds for a dose of healthy fats and protein.

Lunch: Feast on a colorful, nutrient-dense salad with arugula, beets, walnuts, and crumbled feta cheese or a dairy-free alternative. Drizzle with balsamic vinaigrette.

Afternoon Snack: Slice a ripe avocado and sprinkle it with sea salt and black pepper for a satisfying and nourishing snack.

Dinner: Indulge in a grilled salmon fillet or a tofu steak marinated in lemon and herbs. Serve with steamed broccoli and quinoa.

Evening: Sip on a cup of herbal tea before bedtime to aid digestion and promote restful sleep.

Day 3: Cellular Renewal

Morning: Start your day with a glass of warm water infused with fresh mint leaves. Follow with a tropical smoothie made with pineapple, mango, spinach, and a hint of coconut milk.

Mid-Morning Snack: Enjoy a bowl of mixed berries for a burst of antioxidants and natural sweetness.

Lunch: Relish a vibrant and protein-packed salad with mixed greens, grilled shrimp or tempeh, cherry tomatoes, and a zesty lime-cilantro dressing.

Afternoon Snack: Munch on crunchy celery sticks and cherry tomatoes with a light sprinkle of sea salt.

Dinner: Savor a nourishing bowl of vegetable and lentil soup seasoned with turmeric and cumin. Add a side of sautéed spinach or kale for extra greens.

Evening: Conclude your day with a calming cup of chamomile tea to support relaxation and digestion.

This structured meal plan for days 1-3 prioritizes whole, unprocessed foods that are rich in nutrients and antioxidants. It emphasizes hydration, digestive support, and cellular renewal, laying a strong foundation for the rest of your detox journey.

Detoxifying Recipes

To enhance the effectiveness of your physical cleanse, let's explore a selection of detoxifying recipes that align with your meal plan for days 1-3. These recipes are designed to promote detoxification, support weight loss, and nourish your body.

Detox Green Smoothie

Prep Time: 5 minutes, **Total Time:** 5 minutes, **Servings:** 1

Ingredients

- 1 cup spinach
- 1 cup kale
- 1/2 cucumber, peeled and chopped
- 1/2-inch fresh ginger, peeled
- 1 cup water
- Ice cubes (optional)

Instructions

1. In a blender, combine spinach, kale, cucumber, fresh ginger, and water.
2. Blend until smooth, adding ice cubes if desired for a colder smoothie.
3. Pour into a glass and enjoy as a refreshing morning or mid-morning snack.

Nutritional Information (per serving):

Calories: 70	Carbohydrates: 14g	Protein: 3g
Fat: 1g	Fiber: 2g	Sugar: 5g

Detox Salad with Lemon Vinaigrette

Prep Time: 15 minutes, **Total Time:** 15 minutes, **Servings:** 2

Salad Ingredients

- 4 cups mixed greens (e.g., spinach, arugula, and romaine)
- 1 cup cherry tomatoes, halved
- 1 red bell pepper, thinly sliced
- 1/4 cup walnuts, chopped
- 1/4 cup feta cheese (or dairy-free alternative), crumbled
- Lemon Vinaigrette Ingredients:
- 2 tablespoons fresh lemon juice
- 2 tablespoons extra-virgin olive oil
- 1 teaspoon honey (or maple syrup for a vegan option)
- Salt and black pepper to taste

Instructions

1. In a large salad bowl, combine the mixed greens, cherry tomatoes, red bell pepper, walnuts, and feta cheese.
2. In a small jar, whisk together the lemon juice, olive oil, honey (or maple syrup), salt, and black pepper to create the vinaigrette.
3. Drizzle the lemon vinaigrette over the salad and toss to combine.
4. Serve the detox salad for a refreshing and nutrient-rich lunch.

Nutritional Information (per serving):

Calories: 290   Carbohydrates: 16g   Protein: 7g
Fat: 23g   Fiber: 4g   Sugar: 8g

Grilled Salmon with Steamed Broccoli

Prep Time: 10 minutes, **Total Time:** 20 minutes, **Servings:** 2

Ingredients

- 2 salmon fillets (6-8 oz each)
- 2 tablespoons fresh lemon juice
- 1 teaspoon dried oregano
- Salt and black pepper to taste
- 2 cups broccoli florets

Instructions

1. Preheat your grill to medium-high heat.
2. In a small bowl, mix the lemon juice, dried oregano, salt, and black pepper to create a marinade for the salmon.
3. Brush the salmon fillets with the marinade.
4. Place the salmon fillets on the grill and cook for about 4-5 minutes per side, or until the salmon easily flakes with a fork.
5. While the salmon is grilling, steam the broccoli until tender, about 3-4 minutes.
6. Serve the grilled salmon alongside the steamed broccoli for a satisfying and nutritious dinner.

Nutritional Information (per serving):

Calories: 330   Carbohydrates: 7g   Protein: 34g
Fat: 19g   Fiber: 3g   Sugar: 2g

These recipes are just a taste of what you can enjoy during the first three days of your physical cleanse. They prioritize whole, unprocessed ingredients that support detoxification and weight loss while nourishing your body with essential nutrients.

Remember, this is just the beginning of your journey to holistic well-being. The physical cleanse sets the stage for the subsequent phases, each addressing different aspects of your mind, body, and spirit. Stay committed, stay mindful, and embrace the transformative power of the physical cleanse. The days ahead hold the promise of enhanced vitality, clarity, and a deeper connection to your own well-being.

Chapter 7:
Day 4-7: The Mind Reset

Welcome to the next phase of your 14-day mind-body-spirit detox journey. By now, you've begun your physical cleanse, and you're likely starting to feel the benefits of nourishing your body with healthy foods. In the coming days, we'll shift our focus from the physical to the mental aspect of your well-being. The mind is a powerful tool, and its state profoundly influences your overall health. In this chapter, we'll explore how to reset and rejuvenate your mind through mindfulness practices, meditation, and journaling.

Transitioning to the Mind Reset

As you progress through the 14-day mind-body-spirit detox program, the shift from the physical cleanse to the mind reset phase marks a pivotal moment in your holistic well-being journey. It's a time to take the valuable lessons and principles you've learned about nourishing your body and extend them to the realm of your mind. Just as you've been selective about the foods you consume; it is equally important to exercise mindfulness and selectivity in terms of the thoughts and emotions you allow into your mental space.

The mind reset is about beginning a mental cleanse, akin to decluttering your living space or purging your diet of unhealthy foods. It is an opportunity to release the accumulated mental baggage, reduce stress, and ultimately seek balance within yourself. This phase is designed to offer you a chance to reconnect with your inner self, improve your emotional regulation, and cultivate a deep sense of inner peace.

Much like the physical cleanse, the practices introduced in the upcoming days of the mind reset are carefully chosen to align with your holistic health goals. They go beyond just benefiting your mental well-being; they have a positive impact on your overall health. As you transition, embrace this opportunity to declutter your mental space, reduce the burden of stress, and begin a journey of self-discovery. The practices you'll encounter in the days ahead will empower you to take charge of your mind, nurturing it in the same way you've nourished your body. By nurturing your mind, you pave the way for a more profound and lasting sense of holistic well-being.

Mindfulness Practices for Stress Reduction

Mindfulness is a profound and versatile tool for reducing stress and nurturing mental well-being. At its core, mindfulness invites you to be fully present in the current moment, without judgment or preconceived notions. It's about cultivating a heightened awareness of your thoughts, feelings, bodily sensations, and the world around you. During these next four days, we'll delve into a variety of mindfulness practices that you can seamlessly incorporate into your daily routine.

Before we dive into the specific mindfulness practices, let's explore the essence of mindfulness. It's not about emptying your mind or achieving a particular state of tranquility. Instead, mindfulness encourages you to acknowledge and accept your thoughts and emotions without judgment. It's about being present, even when the present moment is challenging or uncomfortable.

Mindfulness is often depicted as a mental muscle that can be trained and strengthened. The more you practice, the more skilled you become at observing your thoughts and emotions from a place of curiosity and non-attachment.

Mindful Breathing

One of the simplest and most effective mindfulness practices is mindful breathing. It's an exercise in focusing your attention on your breath. You can do this anytime and anywhere, making it a versatile tool for stress reduction.

Instructions for Mindful Breathing:

1. Find a quiet and comfortable place to sit or lie down.

2. Close your eyes and take a deep breath in through your nose. Feel your lungs expand and your abdomen rise.

3. Exhale slowly and completely through your mouth.

4. Continue to breathe deeply and rhythmically, paying close attention to each breath. Notice the sensation of the air entering your nostrils, the rise and fall of your chest, and the expansion and contraction of your abdomen.

5. As you breathe, thoughts may naturally arise. That's perfectly normal. Acknowledge them without judgment and gently bring your focus back to your breath.

6. Practicing mindful breathing for just a few minutes can help calm your mind and reduce stress.

Body Scan Meditation

Body scan meditation is another valuable mindfulness practice. It involves directing your attention to various parts of your body, progressively relaxing and releasing tension. It's an excellent practice for becoming more in tune with your physical sensations and letting go of bodily stress.

Instructions for Body Scan Meditation:

1. Find a quiet and comfortable place to sit or lie down.

2. Begin by focusing your attention on your toes. Notice any sensations, tension, or discomfort. Breathe into this area, and as you exhale, release any tension.

3. Slowly shift your attention up to your feet, ankles, and legs, repeating the process of observing sensations and releasing tension.

4. Continue moving up through your body, segment by segment, until you reach the crown of your head.

5. As you progress, remember to acknowledge any thoughts that arise and then return your focus to the body scan.

Guided Meditations

Meditation is indeed a cornerstone of mindfulness, and it holds the power to profoundly impact your mental and emotional well-being. In this section of your 14-day mind-body-spirit detox program, we'll provide you with a collection of guided meditations carefully designed to cater to various aspects of your well-being. These guided meditations are versatile tools that can help you reduce stress, enhance your focus, and improve your emotional regulation.

Meditation, in its essence, is a practice that encourages the stilling of the mind and the exploration of inner awareness. It is a path to a calmer, more focused, and more emotionally resilient self. However, for those new to meditation or even experienced practitioners, the process can sometimes seem daunting, as quieting the mind and finding focus can be challenging. This is where guided meditations come in.

Guided meditations provide a structured and supportive experience. They are often led by a narrator who gently instructs you throughout the meditation. These sessions are designed to help you enter a state of relaxation and inner exploration, making meditation more accessible and enjoyable.

Reducing Stress

Stress is an ever-present factor in our lives, and learning to manage it is crucial for our well-being. Our guided meditation for stress reduction will lead you through a process of relaxation, mindfulness, and self-compassion. By guiding your thoughts and focusing your attention, this meditation will help you unwind and release the accumulated stress of your daily life.

Guided Meditation for Stress Reduction:

1. Find a comfortable, quiet place to sit or lie down.

2. Close your eyes and take slow, deep breaths in and out.

3. Focus on your breath, allowing any thoughts to come and go without judgment.

4. Gradually relax each part of your body, starting from your head and moving down to your toes.

5. Visualize a peaceful scene or location that brings you calmness and serenity.

6. Stay in this state for 10-15 minutes, continuing to focus on your breath.

7. Gently bring your attention back to your surroundings and open your eyes.

8. Take a few moments to reflect on the experience and carry the sense of relaxation with you throughout the day.

Enhancing Focus

In our fast-paced world filled with distractions, enhancing your focus can lead to improved productivity and mental clarity.

The guided meditation for focus is designed to help you hone your attention, sharpen your concentration, and become more present in your daily tasks. This practice will guide you through a journey of self-awareness and mental training, promoting a deeper sense of attentiveness.

Guided Meditation for Enhancing Focus:

1. Find a comfortable sitting position and close your eyes.

2. Take several slow, deep breaths, inhaling fully and exhaling completely.

3. Turn your attention to the natural rhythm of your breath, observing each inhale and exhale.

4. Gently guide your focus to bodily sensations, noticing any tension or relaxation in various areas.

5. Expand awareness to external sounds and sights, observing without judgment or attachment.

6. Practice moments of silence, allowing thoughts to arise and pass without engaging with them.

7. Maintain focused attention for 5-10 minutes before gently bringing your awareness back to the present moment, and slowly opening your eyes.

Improving Emotional Regulation

Emotional regulation is a fundamental skill for managing the ups and downs of life. The guided meditation for emotional regulation will assist you in understanding and managing your emotions more effectively. It will guide you through an exploration of your emotional landscape, fostering a healthier relationship with your feelings and helping you respond to them with greater awareness.

Guided Meditation for Improving Emotional Regulation:

1. Find a comfortable and quiet space to sit or lie down.
2. Close your eyes and take several slow, deep breaths.
3. Gradually pay attention to your body, scanning it for any tension or discomfort.
4. As you notice tension, visualize it releasing and dissolving with each exhale.
5. Shift your focus to the present moment, allowing thoughts and emotions to come and go without judgment.
6. When strong emotions arise, label them gently without dwelling on them, then return your focus to the breath.
7. Continue this practice for 10-15 minutes, gradually increasing the duration over time.
8. Gently bring your awareness back to your surroundings and open your eyes when you feel ready.

Guided meditations are powerful tools of self-discovery and inner transformation. As you embrace these practices, remember that meditation is not about perfection; it's about progress and consistency. The more you engage with these guided meditations, the more you'll notice their positive impact on your mental and emotional well-being. Enjoy the journey as you explore your inner world and cultivate a calmer, more focused, and emotionally resilient self.

Journaling Prompts for Self-Reflection

Journaling is a powerful tool for self-reflection and self-discovery, offering you a private space to explore your thoughts, feelings, and experiences. As you progress through your 14-day mind-body-spirit detox program, journaling will become a valuable ally in your journey toward holistic well-being. Our journaling prompts are designed to guide your reflections, helping you uncover patterns, beliefs, and emotions that may be affecting your mental well-being.

Gratitude Journaling

Practicing gratitude is a simple yet profound way to cultivate a positive mindset and enhance your mental well-being. The act of acknowledging and appreciating the blessings, both big and small, in your life can lead to a greater sense of contentment, joy, and perspective. In this section, we'll delve into the practice of gratitude journaling, which involves answering two key questions:

What are three things you're grateful for today, and why?

Take a moment to reflect on your day and identify three specific things that you're grateful for. These can be events, experiences, people, or aspects of your life. To get the most out of this practice, focus on the details and specifics. Instead of just stating, "I'm grateful for my family," you might say, "I'm grateful for the laughter and warmth of my family during our evening meal."

How did expressing gratitude make you feel? Did it affect your mood or outlook on the day?

After you've identified your sources of gratitude, delve into the emotional aspect of this practice. Consider how acknowledging these blessings made you feel. Did it fill you with joy, contentment, or a sense of abundance? Did it shift your mood or outlook on the day in any way? Reflect on the emotional impact of gratitude and how it influenced your overall well-being.

Emotional Check-In:

An emotional check-in is a mindfulness practice that invites you to pause and tune into your inner world. It's an opportunity to connect with your current emotional state and the sensations in your body. In the rush of daily life, we often neglect our emotional well-being, but this practice encourages you to be present with your feelings. Here, we'll explore two essential questions:

How are you feeling right now, in this moment?

Begin by taking a few deep breaths to center yourself. Then, turn your attention inward and ask yourself how you're feeling at this very moment. This question invites you to identify your emotional state. Are you feeling happy, sad, anxious, content, or any other emotion? It's essential to use accurate and specific labels for your emotions. For example, instead of saying you feel "bad," specify if you feel frustrated, irritated, or disappointed.

Are there any specific emotions or sensations in your body that you can identify?

Emotions are not just mental experiences; they often manifest as physical sensations in your body. This question encourages you to explore the physical dimension of your emotions. Do you notice any sensations, like tension in your shoulders, a knot in your stomach, or a lightness in your chest? Recognizing these bodily cues can provide valuable insights into the physical aspect of your emotional well-being.

Emotional check-ins are an essential practice for increasing self-awareness and emotional regulation. By regularly checking in with your emotions and body, you develop the ability to recognize, accept, and manage your feelings. This practice can help you navigate daily challenges, reduce stress, and promote emotional well-being by allowing you to stay present with your emotions.

Mindfulness Moments:

Mindfulness is about being fully present in the moment, without judgment. It's a practice that can significantly impact your mental well-being by helping you stay connected to the here and now. Mindfulness moments invite you to reflect on your day and recognize instances when you consciously practiced mindfulness. Here, we explore two crucial questions:

Describe a moment today when you practiced mindfulness. How did it make you feel?

Recall a specific moment from your day when you intentionally engaged in mindfulness. This could be during a daily task, a conversation, or a moment of solitude. Describe the situation, what you observed, and how it made you feel. Did you experience a sense of presence, clarity, or calmness during this moment of mindfulness? Reflect on the emotional impact of this practice.

Were there any challenges in staying present, and if so, how did you overcome them?

Mindfulness can sometimes be challenging, especially when distractions, worries, or stressors pull your attention away from the present moment. This question encourages you to consider if you faced any difficulties in staying mindful during the described moment. If you did encounter challenges, how did you overcome them? What strategies or techniques did you employ to return to the state of mindfulness?

Practicing mindfulness moments is a powerful way to enhance your mental well-being. By recognizing and savoring these instances of mindfulness in your day, you reinforce the habit of being present and cultivating a deeper sense of self-awareness. These moments can bring a greater sense of peace, focus, and resilience to your life.

Self-Compassion Exploration:

Self-compassion is an essential component of mental well-being. It involves treating yourself with the same kindness, understanding, and support that you would offer to a close friend in times of difficulty. In this section, we'll explore two aspects of self-compassion:

Reflect on a situation where you may have been self-critical. How might practicing self-compassion have changed your response?

Think back to a recent situation where you may have been overly critical or harsh on yourself. It could be related to a mistake, a personal challenge, or a moment of self-doubt. Reflect on how your response might have been different if you had applied self-compassion. How would offering understanding, kindness, and support to yourself have changed the way you handled the situation? Consider the potential impact on your mental well-being.

Write a self-compassionate letter to yourself, offering understanding and support for any challenges you're currently facing.

In this exercise, you'll compose a letter to yourself as you would to a dear friend facing challenges. Begin by acknowledging the difficulties or struggles you're currently experiencing. Offer words of understanding, empathy, and self-compassion. Be kind to yourself and provide the support and encouragement you would to someone you deeply care about. This exercise can be a profoundly healing practice that nurtures your emotional well-being.

Practicing self-compassion is a powerful means of enhancing your mental health and overall well-being. By recognizing and transforming self-critical thoughts and judgments into self-compassionate responses, you cultivate a more positive and resilient mindset. This practice can contribute to greater emotional regulation, self-acceptance, and inner peace.

Focus and Concentration:

Staying focused and maintaining concentration on a task is a fundamental aspect of mental well-being. It allows you to be more productive, efficient, and engaged with your daily activities. In this section, we explore two questions related to focus and concentration:

Did you encounter any moments today where you felt particularly focused or concentrated on a task?

Reflect on your day and identify instances when you experienced a high level of focus and concentration. This could have been during work, a hobby, reading, or any other activity that required your full attention. Describe the situation and how it made you feel. Recognize the benefits of being fully engaged in the task at hand.

What strategies or techniques helped you maintain your attention?

Maintaining focus and concentration can sometimes be challenging, especially in a world filled with distractions. Consider the strategies or techniques that helped you stay on track during the moments when you were highly focused. Did you use techniques like time management, setting specific goals, eliminating distractions, or taking short breaks? Reflect on the practices that supported your ability to concentrate.

Emotional Regulation:

Emotional regulation is a vital skill for maintaining mental well-being. It involves the ability to identify, understand, and manage your emotions effectively. In this section, we explore two questions related to emotional regulation:

Describe a situation where you experienced a strong emotion. How did you react to it?

Recall a specific situation from your day where you encountered a powerful emotion. It could have been joy, anger, sadness, anxiety, or any other strong feeling. Describe the circumstances, the emotion you felt, and how you initially reacted to it. Consider whether your initial reaction was helpful or not in managing that emotion.

Were there any practices or techniques you used to regulate your emotions during this moment?

Emotions can be intense and sometimes challenging to navigate. Reflect on whether you employed any practices or techniques to regulate your emotions during the described situation. This could include deep breathing, mindfulness, cognitive reframing, or other strategies that helped you manage your emotional response. Recognize the effectiveness of these techniques in enhancing your emotional regulation.

Enhancing emotional regulation is a significant step toward improved mental well-being. It allows you to respond to challenging emotions in a healthy and constructive manner, reducing stress and promoting emotional balance. By identifying the techniques that work best for you, you can develop a more robust emotional regulation toolkit and support your overall mental health

Mind Reset:

The mind reset phase of the program is a transformative journey that holds the promise of enhancing your mental well-being. In this section, we'll explore two questions related to your expectations and hopes for this phase:

As you enter the mind reset phase of the program, what are your expectations or hopes?

Consider what you expect to gain or experience during the mind reset phase. Are you hoping for reduced stress, greater emotional balance, improved focus, or a deeper sense of inner peace? Reflect on the specific outcomes or changes you anticipate as you engage in these practices.

How do you envision your mental well-being improving as you engage in these practices?

Visualize how your mental well-being may evolve and improve as you embrace the mind reset practices. Envision a day in the future when the program is complete. How will your mental state be different from today? How will you feel, think, and respond to life's challenges? Paint a picture of the positive transformation you hope to achieve through these practices.

The mind reset phase is a profound opportunity to nurture your mental well-being and promote holistic health. By setting clear expectations and envisioning the positive impact of these practices, you empower yourself to fully engage in this transformational journey. Remember that the mind is a powerful tool for change, and as you reset and nourish it, you pave the way for a more balanced and peaceful state of being.

Mindful Meditation Experiences:

Guided meditation is a valuable tool for enhancing your mental well-being during the mind reset phase. In this section, we'll explore your experiences with guided meditation and its impact on your mental state and emotional well-being:

Reflect on your experiences with guided meditation. Did you notice any changes in your mental state or emotional well-being after these sessions?

Recall the guided meditation sessions you've engaged in during the mind reset phase. Reflect on how these sessions made you feel both mentally and emotionally. Did you notice any changes in your mental state, such as increased calmness or clarity of thought? How did your emotional well-being evolve after engaging in guided meditation? Recognize the shifts and improvements you observed.

Are there specific meditations that resonate with you more than others?

Consider whether certain guided meditations resonated with you on a deeper level than others. Were there specific themes, techniques, or voices that you found particularly effective or engaging? Identifying the meditations that resonate with you can help you tailor your practice to better suit your needs and preferences.

Inner Clutter:

Mental clutter and distractions can impede your inner peace and well-being. In this section, we'll explore the concept of inner clutter and how to address or release it:

Take a moment to identify any mental clutter or distractions that may be hindering your inner peace. What are they, and how can you address or release them?

Pause and reflect on any mental clutter or distractions that have been occupying your mind. These can be thoughts, worries, fears, or recurring concerns that create mental noise and disrupt your inner peace. Identify them and consider how they affect your mental well-being. Once recognized, explore strategies to address or release these distractions. This could involve mindfulness, journaling, or other techniques that help declutter your mind and restore inner peace.

Acknowledging and addressing inner clutter is a vital step in your journey toward mental well-being. By identifying the distractions and finding ways to release them, you create space for clarity, focus, and a greater sense of inner peace. This process allows you to fully engage in the mind reset practices and experience their profound impact on your holistic health.

Journey Insights:

The mind reset phase of the program is a time of introspection and self-discovery. In this section, we'll explore the insights and personal revelations you've gained about your mental and emotional well-being:

As you reflect on the past few days, what insights or personal revelations have you gained about your mental and emotional well-being?

Consider the experiences, practices, and reflections of the past few days. What insights or personal revelations have emerged about your mental and emotional well-being? Have you discovered patterns in your thoughts or emotions? Have you found new ways to reduce stress or enhance emotional regulation? Reflect on these insights and personal revelations that are shaping your journey.

How do you envision these insights shaping your journey towards holistic health?

Envision how these newfound insights will influence your ongoing journey towards holistic health. How will they inform your approach to nurturing your mind and emotional well-being? Think about the positive changes and growth that these insights may bring to your holistic health and well-being.

The mind reset phase is not only about reducing stress and enhancing emotional balance but also about gaining a deeper understanding of your mental and emotional landscape. Your insights are valuable steppingstones on this path, guiding you toward a more peaceful and balanced state of being as you progress through the program.

Embracing the Mind Reset phase of your 14-day mind-body-spirit detox program is an opportunity for deep self-exploration and transformation. Journaling is your companion on this journey, providing a safe space for you to articulate your thoughts and emotions, celebrate your achievements, and address challenges. As you embrace this phase, remember that you're nourishing your mind just as you nourish your body, contributing to a more balanced, peaceful, and self-aware self. Continue to explore your inner landscape with curiosity and compassion.

115

Chapter 8:
Day 8-11: Nourishing the Spirit

In the second half of your 14-day mind-body-spirit detox journey, we shift our focus towards the spiritual dimension of holistic well-being. Days 8 to 11 are dedicated to nurturing your spirit, connecting with inner purpose and meaning, and encouraging self-reflection on your life's journey.

The spiritual dimension of well-being encompasses our sense of purpose, connection to something greater than ourselves, and our innermost beliefs and values. It transcends religious affiliation and dogma, as it is a deeply personal and subjective aspect of our existence. It is about seeking meaning and purpose in life, connecting with the universe or a higher power, living by our values and beliefs, and experiencing moments of transcendence.

As we start this phase of the program, we will explore practices and activities that promote a sense of purpose, connection, and inner growth. These practices can help you navigate the spiritual dimension and enrich your holistic health.

Nurturing the Spirit: Embracing the Spiritual Dimension of Well-Being

In our fast-paced, materialistic world, we often find ourselves preoccupied with the demands of daily life, leaving little room to nurture our spiritual dimension. However, the spiritual aspect of well-being is an integral part of holistic health, contributing significantly to our overall vitality and sense of fulfillment. Nurturing the spirit involves engaging in practices and activities that foster a deeper connection with our inner selves, a sense of purpose, and an enhanced understanding of our place in the grand tapestry of existence. Here, we explore various practices that can help you nurture the spiritual dimension of your well-being:

Gratitude: The Power of Appreciation

Cultivating gratitude is a powerful spiritual practice. It involves acknowledging and appreciating the blessings, both big and small, in our lives. In the hustle and bustle of modern living, it's easy to become ensnared by a mindset of scarcity, where we perpetually focus on what we lack. Practicing gratitude is like a gentle shift in perspective, redirecting our gaze from scarcity to abundance. It fosters contentment and a profound sense of fulfillment, reminding us of the richness of our existence.

Activity: Consider starting a gratitude journal, where you document three things, you're grateful for each day, along with the reasons for your gratitude. Reflect on how this practice makes you feel and how it influences your outlook on life.

Journaling: The Path to Self-Exploration

Keeping a journal is a time-honored means of self-reflection and spiritual exploration. It offers an intimate space to explore your thoughts, feelings, and experiences, granting your insight into your inner world and promoting personal growth. Journaling can be a therapeutic journey into your consciousness, providing clarity about your beliefs, values, and emotional landscapes.

Activity: Begin journaling as part of your daily routine. You can start with simple entries about your experiences and feelings. Gradually, delve deeper into your inner world, exploring your goals, dreams, and the values that underpin your life.

Meditation: The Gateway to Transcendence

Meditation is a versatile and profound practice that can lead to deep spiritual experiences. It allows you to connect with your inner self, delve into your thoughts and emotions, and experience moments of transcendence and clarity. Meditation can be a source of serenity and inner peace, fostering a deeper understanding of your inner world.

Activity: If you're new to meditation, start with short daily sessions. Find a quiet and comfortable space, close your eyes, and focus on your breath. As you grow more comfortable with this practice, explore different meditation techniques, such as loving-kindness meditation or mindfulness meditation.

Mindfulness: Embracing the Present Moment

Mindfulness is a practice deeply rooted in the spiritual dimension of well-being. It involves being fully present in the moment, without judgment. Mindfulness enables you to appreciate the beauty of the present, fostering a deeper sense of connection and inner peace. It encourages you to savor the simple moments in life and rediscover the sense of wonder in the world around you.

Activity: Incorporate mindfulness into your daily life by consciously engaging in routine activities. For example, when eating, focus solely on the flavors and textures of your food. When walking, become aware of each step. Through these practices, you can develop a heightened sense of presence.

Nature Connection: Finding Awe and Interconnectedness

Spending time in nature is a deeply spiritual practice. Nature's grandeur, from towering mountains to delicate wildflowers, can inspire a sense of awe and wonder. In the embrace of nature, you can connect with the larger universe and the intricate web of life. You may find that moments spent in nature provide clarity and insight, strengthening your spiritual connection.

Activity: Regularly dedicate time to connect with nature. This could be a leisurely walk in the park, a hike through the woods, or simply sitting in your garden. Use these moments to reflect on your place in the world and the interconnectedness of all living beings.

Acts of Kindness: Nurturing Compassion and Purpose

Engaging in acts of kindness and service to others is deeply spiritual. It allows you to connect with your compassion and empathy, fostering a profound sense of purpose and fulfillment. Acts of kindness promote a sense of interconnectedness and mutual support, reminding us of the beauty in our shared humanity.

Activity: Integrate small acts of kindness into your daily life. It could be as simple as offering a smile to a stranger, helping a colleague, or volunteering your time to support a charitable cause. These acts, no matter how modest, contribute to your spiritual growth.

Finding Purpose: Aligning with Your Deepest Values

Finding purpose is a central aspect of the spiritual dimension. It involves aligning your actions with your deepest values and beliefs. Discovering your purpose is a journey of self-discovery, during which you explore the profound questions about your existence and your role in the world. It's about creating a meaningful and fulfilling life that resonates with your innermost aspirations.

Activity: Reflect on your values and beliefs. Explore what truly matters to you and what you'd like to contribute to the world. As you uncover your purpose, consider how you can align your daily actions and decisions with this guiding star.

Nurturing the spirit is a transformative journey that takes time and patience. The practices mentioned above are not mere activities; they are gateways to profound experiences and inner growth. By consistently incorporating these practices into your life, you can deepen your spiritual connection and foster a sense of purpose and inner peace that contributes significantly to your holistic health and well-being.

The journey toward holistic well-being is a remarkable voyage. It is not solely about reaching a specific destination but also about the path you have traveled, the experiences you have encountered, and the wisdom you have amassed along the way. During days 8 to 11 of your 14-day mind-body-spirit detox program, you will have the opportunity to engage in self-reflection on your life's journey. This period of deep spiritual practice allows you to contemplate where you've been, where you stand now, and where you aspire to go. As you partake in practices that connect you with your inner purpose and meaning, consider these essential aspects of self-reflection:

Past Experiences

Begin by reflecting on the past experiences that have significantly impacted your spiritual dimension. These experiences can range from the joyous and uplifting to the arduous and challenging. Delve into the events and moments that have left an indelible mark on your spiritual journey. How have these experiences influenced your sense of purpose and meaning in life? What wisdom have you garnered from both the moments of celebration and those that presented you with obstacles to overcome?

Values and Beliefs

Take a closer look at the values and beliefs that serve as the compass for your life's journey. These principles guide your daily actions and decisions, whether consciously or unconsciously. Consider how your values and beliefs align with your spiritual dimension. How do they enhance your sense of purpose and meaning, and what role do they play in fostering your holistic well-being? Reflect on how these values have evolved and developed throughout your life.

Transcendent Moments

Explore moments in your life when you experienced a sense of transcendence or connection with something greater than yourself. These moments may manifest as a deep connection with nature, an overwhelming sense of awe in the presence of art, or a profound spiritual experience. Reflect on how these moments have influenced your spiritual well-being and your overall holistic health. How have they changed your perspective on life and your place within the universe?

Acts of Kindness

Review the acts of kindness and service to others that you have undertaken. Consider how these actions have contributed to your sense of purpose and fulfillment. Acts of kindness have the remarkable ability to connect you with your innate compassion and empathy, fostering a deeper understanding of your role in the world and your interconnectedness with all living beings. How have your experiences in helping others illuminated the path toward your fulfillment?

Gratitude

Engage in the practice of gratitude, taking time to reflect on the things you are grateful for in your spiritual dimension. The art of gratitude can shift your focus from scarcity to abundance, fostering contentment and a profound sense of fulfillment. Contemplate how your practice of gratitude influences your perception of life, your sense of abundance, and your overall well-being.

Future Aspirations

As you venture forward, envision the future and how you intend to nurture your spiritual dimension. What practices and activities will you continue to explore to enrich your holistic well-being? Consider the spiritual journey you aspire to undertake, drawing inspiration from the transformative experiences of the past eight days. Chart a course that aligns with your unique values, beliefs, and aspirations. How do you foresee your spiritual dimension evolving in the days, months, and years to come?

As we journey through the spiritual dimension of holistic well-being on days 8 to 11, remember that it's a deeply personal and subjective aspect of our existence. There is no one-size-fits-all approach, and your spiritual journey is unique to you. Embrace the practices, reflect on your life's journey, and allow yourself to connect with your inner purpose and meaning in a way that resonates with your heart and soul. It's a profound phase of your 14-day mind-body-spirit detox program, where you'll experience the deep and transformative effects of nurturing your spirit.

Chapter 9:
Day 12-14: The Holistic Fusion

In the final stretch of your 14-day mind-body-spirit detox program, we bring together the physical, mental, and spiritual elements to create a holistic fusion. These last three days are dedicated to integrating everything you've learned and experienced, allowing you to fully embrace the benefits of holistic living and transformation.

Holistic living is about recognizing that well-being is not just the absence of illness but a state of thriving in all dimensions of your life. It's the harmonious fusion of the physical, mental, and spiritual aspects that makes this possible. To achieve this fusion, we provide a comprehensive daily plan that combines fasting, mindfulness, and spiritual reflection. This fusion will highlight the transformative effects of your holistic journey and inspire you to continue nurturing your well-being.

The Holistic Fusion Plan

Day 12: Mindful Eating

Morning: A Breath of Fresh Start

As the sun begins to rise and a new day unfolds, you'll commence your morning with a mindfulness meditation. This practice sets a positive tone and primes your mind for the day ahead. Your focus should be directed toward the sensations of your breath. Observe the gentle rhythm of inhaling and exhaling, recognizing the life-sustaining energy it provides you. Inhale clarity and exhale any lingering disturbances. Allow the meditative stillness to envelop you, cultivating a sense of peace that will accompany you throughout the day.

Breakfast: A Nourishing Beginning

Break your fast with a nourishing and mindful meal. Choose your food mindfully, considering how it nourishes your body. With your plate before you, take a moment to express gratitude for the nourishment it offers. As you take each bite, savor the flavors and textures that dance upon your palate. Pay attention to the way your body responds to this nourishing sustenance. How does it make you feel physically and emotionally? Allow your senses to be fully present and engaged as you appreciate this experience of mindful eating.

Mid-Morning: A Pause for Presence

In the mid-morning, pause for a moment of mindfulness. Find a quiet space where you can ground yourself in the present moment. Connect with your breath, as it is your anchor to the "now." Even amid a busy day, these few minutes of mindfulness can help you maintain a sense of tranquility and awareness.

Lunch: The Art of Appreciation

As you break for lunch, be mindful of the meal you have prepared. Whether it's a sandwich, salad, or any other creation, approach it with gratitude. Express your thanks for the nourishment you are about to receive. Take note of your body's hunger and fullness cues as you enjoy your meal. Being attentive to these signals guides you toward eating in alignment with your body's needs, ensuring both nourishment and fulfillment.

Afternoon: A Nature Embrace

In the afternoon, venture out for a walk in the open air. Whether you find yourself surrounded by the bustling sounds of the city or the serene whispers of nature, take a moment to connect with your environment. Immerse yourself in the beauty of the world around you. Observe the vibrancy of life, whether it's the vivid colors of urban landscapes or the serene majesty of the natural world. The afternoon walks, combined with mindfulness, allows you to recharge your spirit and maintain your focus on the present.

Dinner: Reflecting on the Nourishing Journey

As the day winds down, prepare for a mindful dinner. This meal serves not only to nourish your body but to provide an opportunity for reflection. Sit down to your dinner plate, fully engaged and present in the moment. Reflect on the journey you've experienced and the changes you've experienced. Mindful eating has a profound impact on your holistic well-being, enhancing your connection to nourishment and promoting a healthier relationship with food.

Evening: Journaling the Essence of Mindful Eating

In the evening, dedicate a moment to journal about your experience with mindful eating throughout the day. Consider how this practice has impacted your overall well-being. Did you notice changes in the way you related to food or your body? Reflect on the sensory experiences and how they enhanced your connection to nourishment. Journaling is a valuable tool for self-reflection and self-discovery, providing insights into your holistic health journey.

Day 12 is a celebration of the union between nourishment and mindfulness. It's an opportunity to foster a deeper connection with the sustenance that fuels your body and to appreciate each bite as a gift to your well-being. Mindful eating offers a gateway to nurturing the body, mind, and spirit through your relationship with food, marking another profound step on your path to holistic well-being.

Day 13: Spiritual Connection

Morning: The Gratitude Meditation

Begin your day with a gratitude meditation, expressing thanks for the remarkable journey you've undertaken. Take a few moments to sit in stillness, breathing deeply and deliberately. Inhale gratitude for the experiences, lessons, and growth you've encountered. Exhale any remaining doubts or uncertainties. As you immerse yourself in the feelings of gratitude, you'll recognize how far you've come in your quest for holistic well-being.

Breakfast: A Meal with Spiritual Intention

The morning meal is more than a simple breaking of the fast; it is a conscious and spiritually aligned experience. As you select your nourishing foods, set an intention for the day. This intention should encompass mindfulness, compassion, and alignment with your core values and beliefs. Let the process of choosing, preparing, and eating your breakfast be a sacred act that honors your connection to your spiritual dimension.

Mid-Morning: The Deepening Meditation

Engage in a session of mindful meditation in the mid-morning. This practice is not only a moment of stillness but also a journey to deepen your connection with the spiritual dimension. Find a quiet and peaceful space where you can comfortably sit or lie down. Begin with a few deep breaths, centering yourself. As you delve into your meditation, allow yourself to become more aware of your inner self and the interconnectedness of all living beings. Feel the resonance with something greater than yourself and cultivate a profound sense of peace.

Lunch: A Conscious Culinary Experience

Your lunch should be a meal that deeply aligns with your values and beliefs. Reflect on how your dietary choices can impact your spiritual well-being. Select foods that honor your spiritual path and values, such as plant-based options or foods that are locally sourced and sustainable. As you eat, be mindful of the connection between your food and the nourishment of your soul.

Afternoon: Nature's Embrace and Contemplation

Nature, in its serene and boundless beauty, serves as a gateway to the spiritual dimension. Spend your afternoon immersed in the natural world, whether you find yourself amidst the grandeur of the outdoors or simply within the embrace of an urban park. Take time to connect with the universe or higher power that resonates with you. Engage in contemplation and offer gratitude for the interconnectedness of all life. In nature's presence, recognize the sacredness of the world and your place within it.

Dinner: Sharing Spiritual Nourishment

Your evening meal offers a chance to share a spiritually nourishing experience with loved ones. Gather with friends or family and create an atmosphere that fosters a sense of oneness and connection. As you dine together, reflect on the interconnectedness of your lives and the spiritual growth you've cultivated on this journey. Conversations can revolve around the experiences of the day, the wisdom you've gathered, and the spiritual connections you've felt.

Evening: Journaling the Soul's Connection

As your day comes to a close, write in your journal about the spiritual connection you've experienced throughout the day. Reflect on how this connection has impacted your sense of purpose and meaning. Explore the profound experiences, insights, and feelings you've encountered as you've deepened your spiritual connection. This self-reflection is an invaluable practice that aids in your continued growth and transformation.

Day 13 is a remarkable step in your holistic well-being journey, where you nourish your soul and expand your connection to the spiritual dimension. As you progress through the practices of gratitude, intention, meditation, and conscious dining, you'll cultivate a deeper understanding of your spiritual path and how it contributes to your holistic health.

Day 14: Mind, Body, Spirit Integration

Morning: The Holistic Fusion Meditation

Begin the final day with a holistic fusion meditation. In the quiet of the morning, find a comfortable and serene space. As you sit in stillness, visualize the profound harmony between your mind, body, and spirit. Picture each element working in unison, like the notes of a beautiful symphony, producing a harmonious and balanced existence. This meditation sets the tone for the day, encouraging you to embrace the holistic fusion of your well-being.

Breakfast: A Balanced and Mindful Start

Break your fast on the last day with a meal that embodies the integration of the three dimensions of well-being: mind, body, and spirit. Your breakfast should be a conscious and balanced combination of nourishing foods that represent the holistic lifestyle you've cultivated. As you savor each bite, take a moment to appreciate the interconnectedness of your well-being.

Mid-Morning: Mind-Body-Spirit Connection

Engage in a mindful meditation during the mid-morning, focusing on the unity and integration of the mind, body, and spirit. Let this meditation reinforce the bond that you've nurtured among these core dimensions of well-being. It's an opportunity to become more aware of the balance you've achieved.

Lunch: An Essence of Holistic Living

The midday meal should embody the essence of holistic living. As you consume your lunch, reflect on the incredible journey you've undertaken and the profound transformations you've experienced. The meal represents the culmination of your efforts to nourish your entire being—mind, body, and spirit.

Afternoon: Nature's Celebration

Spend the afternoon in the embrace of nature, celebrating the interconnectedness of all life. Whether you're surrounded by lush forests, serene water bodies, or an urban park, the focus is on recognizing the oneness of existence. This time in nature reinforces your deep sense of purpose and connection with the world around you.

Dinner: A Holistic Fusion Meal

As the sun sets on this extraordinary day, partake in a holistic fusion dinner. This can be a shared experience with loved ones or a reflective solitary meal. Let the experience symbolize your commitment to holistic well-being. The foods on your plate should represent the harmony and balance you've achieved.

Evening: Journaling the Lasting Benefits

In the evening, as your 14-day detox program concludes, write in your journal about the holistic fusion you've embraced and the enduring benefits it has brought to your life. Reflect on the transformations, insights, and experiences you've gained throughout this remarkable journey. Your journal is a testament to your commitment to holistic living and well-being.

As you move through these final three days of your detox program, you'll experience the beauty of holistic living and transformation. The physical, mental, and spiritual elements come together to create a symphony of well-being. Holistic living is a continuous journey, and these days will inspire you to maintain and further develop your holistic health. The benefits of holistic living extend beyond the program, enhancing your overall quality of life and bringing a profound sense of fulfillment. Congratulations on your commitment to well-being and holistic living!

Chapter 10:
Life After the Detox

As you approach the end of your 14-day mind-body-spirit detox program, you may be wondering how to transition to a long-term holistic lifestyle that sustains the benefits you've gained during this transformative journey. In this final chapter, we'll guide you on how to make the shift from detox to everyday life while maintaining and nurturing your well-being. We'll explore strategies for integrating intermittent fasting into your daily routine and discuss how to continue reaping the rewards of a holistic approach.

Transitioning to a Long-Term Holistic Lifestyle

The 14-day mind-body-spirit detox program you've undertaken is a profound step toward nurturing your holistic well-being. It's a transformative journey that offers insights into the interplay of your mind, body, and spirit. As you transition to a long-term holistic lifestyle, the essence is to translate these experiences and discoveries into daily conscious choices. Here's a guide to making this transition a sustainable and enriching part of your life:

Set Clear Intentions:

The first step in your transition to a long-term holistic lifestyle is to define your intentions and goals. What aspects of your well-being do you want to maintain or enhance? Be specific about what you hope to achieve. Whether it's improved physical health, enhanced mental clarity, or a deeper spiritual connection, having clear intentions will act as your guiding light. These intentions will help you make daily choices that are in alignment with your overarching goals.

Routine Integration:

The routines and practices you've established during the detox program can and should be integrated into your daily life. Continuity in these practices is key to maintaining and strengthening your mental and spiritual well-being. Engage in mindfulness, meditation, and journaling as part of your daily routine. These practices have shown to be profoundly transformative, and consistency in incorporating them will deepen their impact over time.

Mindful Eating:

One of the most significant and enduring aspects of your detox program is the principle of mindful eating. Continue to carry this practice forward. Approach your meals with intention and mindfulness. Savor the flavors and textures of your food, being present with each bite. Pay attention to your body's hunger and fullness cues and make informed choices that nourish your body and align with your values. The practice of mindful eating supports not only your physical health but also a harmonious mind and spirit.

Spiritual Connection:

The spiritual practices you've engaged in, whether they involve gratitude, meditation, spending time in nature, or any other form of connection, should remain a constant in your life. Continue to nurture your spiritual connection by integrating these practices into your daily routine. Consistency is key to deepening this aspect of your well-being over time. Keep in mind that spirituality is a personal and evolving journey, so allow these practices to grow and evolve with you.

Support Network:

Share your holistic living journey with friends and family. Seek their understanding and support. Having a community that shares your values and embraces a holistic lifestyle can significantly impact your commitment and success. It's not only about receiving support but also about inspiring and influencing those around you to embrace well-being holistically.

Reflect and Adjust:

Holistic living is dynamic and ever evolving. Your needs, goals, and priorities may change over time. Regularly reflect on your progress and be open to adjusting your approach as needed. Don't be afraid to evolve your practices and routines to align with your current state and aspirations. Flexibility and self-awareness are key components of sustaining a holistic lifestyle.

As you embrace a long-term holistic lifestyle, remember that it's a continuous journey. The 14-day detox program is just the beginning. By making conscious choices each day and integrating the practices and insights you've gained, you can enjoy enduring well-being and lead a more fulfilling, balanced, and harmonious life. Your holistic well-being is not a destination but a path you walk every day.

Maintaining the Benefits of the Detox Program:

The 14-day detox program you've just completed isn't just a self-contained experience; it's a portal to a lifestyle of sustained well-being. To maintain the program's invaluable benefits and continue your journey toward holistic living, you'll want to integrate several key practices and principles into your daily life:

Mindful Awareness:

Stay Present: The foundation of your well-being is mindful awareness. Continue to cultivate mindfulness by staying present in your daily life. Be conscious of your thoughts, emotions, and bodily sensations. Awareness allows you to understand how you react to various stimuli and situations, and it's a powerful tool for reducing stress and promoting your overall well-being.

Mindfulness Techniques: Continue to employ mindfulness techniques to enhance your daily life. These may include mindful breathing exercises, body scans, and walking meditations. In moments of stress or uncertainty, these techniques can guide you back to a state of calm and centeredness.

Nourishing Practices:

Mindful Eating: The practice of mindful eating has likely left a lasting impression on you. It's not just a part of the detox program; it's a practice that can offer sustained well-being.

Approach each meal with intention and presence. Savor the flavors, textures, and nourishment your food provides. Pay attention to your body's hunger and fullness cues and make food choices that align with your well-being goals. Mindful eating isn't just a mealtime ritual; it's a way of relating to food and nourishment that can benefit you in perpetuity.

Gratitude Journaling: Continue your journey of gratitude through journaling. Regularly record the things you're grateful for, both big and small. This practice has the power to shift your focus from what you lack to what you have, fostering contentment and a sense of abundance in your daily life. Writing down your gratitude can be a daily or weekly ritual, offering a moment of reflection and positivity.

Intermittent Fasting:

Embrace a Long-Term Lifestyle Choice: Intermittent fasting isn't just a part of the detox program; it's a lifestyle choice that can have profound impacts on your well-being. Start by selecting a fasting schedule that fits seamlessly into your daily routine. Many people begin with the 16/8 method, which involves fasting for 16 hours and eating during an 8-hour window. As your body adapts and you become more comfortable with fasting, you can gradually increase your fasting window or experiment with other fasting protocols, such as the 5:2 or the 24-hour fast.

Health Benefits: Intermittent fasting can bring about various health benefits, including improved metabolic health, better blood sugar control, weight management, and enhanced brain function. Remember that fasting isn't about deprivation; it's about optimizing your nourishment patterns to support your overall well-being. Consult with a healthcare professional before making significant changes to your fasting routine, especially if you have underlying health conditions or concerns.

Wellness Integration:

The culmination of the detox program is not the end; it's the start of a lifelong journey toward sustained well-being. The lessons and practices you've embraced are tools that you can use every day to cultivate a life of balance, harmony, and fulfillment. By staying present with mindful awareness, nourishing your mind, body, and spirit through ongoing practices, and continuing the beneficial aspects of intermittent fasting, you're creating the foundation for a life that thrives on holistic well-being. Remember that well-being is not a destination; it's a path that you walk each day.

Strategies for Incorporating Intermittent Fasting into Daily Life: A Lifelong Commitment to Well-Being

The practice of intermittent fasting is a valuable tool you've discovered on your journey to holistic well-being. It's not just a temporary phase; it's a long-term lifestyle choice that can promote health, balance, and sustained well-being. Here are some strategies to help you seamlessly incorporate intermittent fasting into your daily routine:

Choose a Fasting Schedule:

Selecting the right fasting schedule is pivotal. Choose a fasting method that harmonizes with your lifestyle and personal preferences. Some common options include:

- **16:8 Method:** This involves fasting for 16 hours and eating during an 8-hour window. You can adapt the eating window to your daily schedule.

- **5:2 Method:** In this approach, you consume a regular diet for five days and limit your calorie intake to about 500-600 calories on two non-consecutive days.

- **OMAD** (One Meal a Day): As the name suggests, this method involves eating one substantial meal during a 1-2-hour window, with a full fast for the rest of the day.

Experiment with these methods and find the one that aligns most seamlessly with your daily commitments and personal well-being goals.

Gradual Progression:

If you're new to intermittent fasting, consider a gradual progression. Start with a fasting window that feels accessible and gradually extend it as your body adapts. Perhaps begin with a 12-hour fast, then progress to 14 hours, and eventually to the 16:8 method. Slow and steady progression helps your body adapt and makes the transition into intermittent fasting smoother.

Remember that the goal of intermittent fasting is to create a sustainable practice that supports your holistic well-being. Listen to your body and make adjustments as needed.

Hydration and Nutrition:

During fasting periods, it's crucial to stay hydrated. Drink plenty of water, herbal teas, or black coffee to quench your thirst and maintain your well-being. These beverages can also help reduce hunger sensations and keep you energized during fasting periods.

When you break your fast, prioritize nutrient-dense, balanced meals. Consider incorporating a variety of whole foods, including vegetables, lean proteins, healthy fats, and complex carbohydrates. These meals should nourish your body, support your energy levels, and align with your holistic living goals.

Listen to Your Body:

Intuitive eating is a significant aspect of intermittent fasting. Pay close attention to your body's hunger and fullness cues. Intermittent fasting should not lead to deprivation or discomfort. It's about nourishing your body within a specific time window that works best for you. When you're genuinely hungry, enjoy your meals mindfully and appreciate the nourishment they provide.

Fasting with Purpose:

Use your fasting periods as an opportunity for purposeful reflection and nourishment of your mind and spirit. Incorporate mindfulness, gratitude, or meditation into your fasting practices. These practices can deepen the holistic benefits of intermittent fasting by supporting mental clarity, reducing stress, and fostering a sense of connection and well-being.

Your journey toward holistic well-being doesn't end when your detox program concludes; it continues as an integral part of your daily life. By embracing intermittent fasting and combining it with mindful awareness, nourishing practices, and a deep sense of purpose, you'll continue to experience the transformative benefits that holistic living offers. It's not a destination; it's an ongoing journey, a lifelong commitment to well-being and self-awareness. Embrace it with an open heart, set clear intentions, and make conscious choices every day.

Chapter 11:

Holistic Recipes for Continued Wellness

In your journey to embrace a holistic lifestyle, nourishing your body with wholesome, nutrient-dense foods plays a vital role. This chapter offers a collection of holistic recipes that you can incorporate into your daily life, supporting the well-being of your body, mind, and spirit. From breakfast to dinner and even snacks, these recipes emphasize the importance of using natural, whole ingredients to enhance your holistic health.

Breakfast Recipes:

These holistic snack ideas are designed to provide nourishment for your body, mind, and spirit. By selecting whole, nutrient-dense ingredients, you are supporting your holistic well-being. Remember that holistic living is not about strict rules but about making conscious, nourishing choices that align with your body and your well-being goals. Enjoy these snacks as part of your journey toward continued wellness!

Detox Green Smoothie

Prep Time: 10 minutes, **Total Time:** 10 minutes, **Servings:** 2

Ingredients

- 2 cups of fresh spinach leaves
- 1 ripe banana
- 1 cup of unsweetened almond milk
- 2 tablespoons of chia seeds
- 1/2 cup of mixed berries (e.g., strawberries, blueberries, raspberries)
- A sprinkle of granola

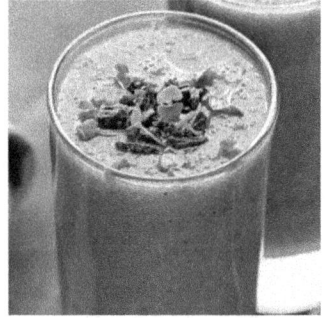

Instructions

1. In a blender, combine the fresh spinach, banana, and unsweetened almond milk. Blend until you have a smooth, vibrant green mixture.
2. Pour the green smoothie into bowls.
3. Top the smoothie with mixed berries and a sprinkle of granola for added texture and crunch.
4. Add chia seeds for an extra nutritional boost.
5. Serve immediately and enjoy your nutrient-packed green smoothie bowl!

Nutritional Information (per serving):

Calories: 300
Fiber: 12g
Saturated Fat: 1.5g
Vitamin A: 120%
Iron: 15%

Protein: 10g
Sugars: 18g
Cholesterol: 0mg
Vitamin C: 80%

Carbohydrates: 40g
Fat: 12g
Sodium: 150mg
Calcium: 30%

Chia Pudding

Prep Time: 5 minutes (plus overnight chilling), **Total Time:** Overnight (or at least 4 hours), **Servings:** 2

Ingredients

- 1/4 cup chia seeds
- 1 cup unsweetened almond milk
- 1 tablespoon honey (or maple syrup for a vegan option)
- Fresh fruit of your choice (e.g., sliced strawberries, kiwi, or blueberries)

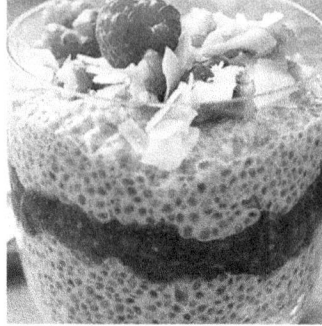

Instructions

1. In a bowl, combine chia seeds and almond milk. Stir well to prevent clumps.
2. Add honey or your chosen sweetener and mix thoroughly.
3. Cover the bowl and refrigerate it overnight (or for at least 4 hours) to allow the chia seeds to absorb the liquid and form a pudding-like consistency.
4. In the morning, divide the chia pudding into two servings.
5. Top each serving with fresh fruit, such as sliced strawberries, kiwi, or blueberries.
6. Enjoy your nutritious and satisfying chia pudding for a wholesome start to your day.

Nutritional Information (per serving, without fruit toppings):

Calories: 210
Fiber: 10g
Saturated Fat: 1g
Calcium: 25%

Protein: 6g
Sugars: 6g
Cholesterol: 0mg
Iron: 10%

Carbohydrates: 20g
Fat: 12g
Sodium: 100mg

Overnight Oats

Prep Time: 5 minutes (plus overnight chilling), **Total Time:** Overnight (or at least 4 hours), **Servings:** 2

Ingredients

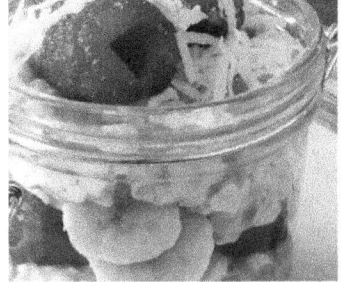

- 1 cup rolled oats
- 1 1/2 cups unsweetened almond milk
- 1/2 cup Greek yogurt
- 2 tablespoons honey (or maple syrup)
- 1/2 cup mixed berries (e.g., blueberries, raspberries)

Instructions

1. In a container or jar, combine rolled oats, almond milk, Greek yogurt, and honey. Stir well to combine all the ingredients thoroughly.
2. Seal the container and refrigerate it overnight (or for at least 4 hours) to allow the oats to soak and soften.
3. In the morning, give the oats a good stir.
4. Divide the overnight oats into two servings.
5. Top each serving with mixed berries or your preferred toppings.
6. Your protein and fiber-packed overnight oats are ready to be enjoyed as a satisfying breakfast.

Nutritional Information (per serving, without additional toppings):

Calories: 320
Fiber: 8g
Saturated Fat: 1g
Calcium: 25%

Protein: 12g
Sugars: 14g
Cholesterol: 5mg
Iron: 2%

Carbohydrates: 50g
Fat: 8g
Sodium: 100mg

Quinoa Salad

Prep Time: 15 minutes, **Total Time:** 30 minutes (if quinoa needs to be cooked), **Servings:** 2

Ingredients

- 1 cup cooked quinoa
- 1/2 cup diced cucumber
- 1/2 cup cherry tomatoes, halved
- 1/2 cup bell peppers (assorted colors), diced
- Fresh herbs (e.g., basil, mint, or cilantro), chopped
- Lemon-tahini dressing (pre-made or homemade)

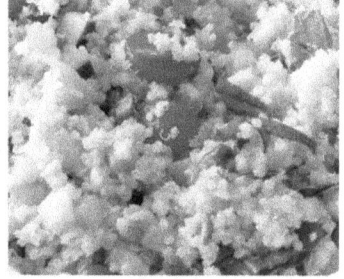

Instructions

1. If not pre-cooked, prepare quinoa according to the package instructions. Allow it to cool before using in the salad.
2. In a large bowl, combine cooked quinoa, diced cucumber, halved cherry tomatoes, diced bell peppers, and a generous amount of fresh, chopped herbs.
3. Drizzle the salad with lemon-tahini dressing and toss to combine all the ingredients.
4. Serve the quinoa salad as a refreshing and nutrient-packed lunch option.

Nutritional Information (per serving):

Calories: 350	Protein: 10g	Carbohydrates: 50g
Fiber: 8g	Sugars: 4g	Fat: 14g
Saturated Fat: 2g	Cholesterol: 0mg	Sodium: 220mg
Vitamin A: 20%	Vitamin C: 90%	Calcium: 10%
Iron: 20%		

Vegetable Stir-Fry

Prep Time: 15 minutes, **Total Time:** 30 minutes, **Servings:** 2

Ingredients

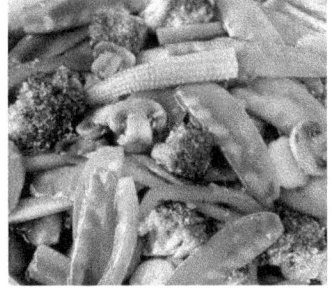

- A mix of colorful veggies (e.g., bell peppers, broccoli, carrots, snap peas)
- Tofu or tempeh, cubed
- Homemade stir-fry sauce (made from ingredients like soy sauce, ginger, garlic, and sesame oil)

Instructions

1. Cut the tofu or tempeh into bite-sized cubes.
2. Heat a non-stick skillet or wok over medium-high heat. Add a small amount of oil, then add the tofu or tempeh cubes and cook until golden brown. Remove from the skillet and set aside.
3. In the same skillet, add a little more oil if needed, then stir-fry your choice of colorful veggies. Start with harder veggies (e.g., carrots, broccoli), and add softer ones (e.g., bell peppers, snap peas) later.
4. Once the veggies are crisp-tender, return the cooked tofu or tempeh to the skillet.
5. Pour the homemade stir-fry sauce over the tofu, tempeh, and veggies. Stir well and let it cook for a couple of minutes until everything is well coated and heated through.
6. Serve your nutrient-rich vegetable stir-fry as a delicious and satisfying lunch.

Nutritional Information (per serving, without rice or noodles):

Calories: 250	Protein: 14g	Carbohydrates: 15g
Fiber: 5g	Sugars: 7g	Fat: 15g
Saturated Fat: 2g	Cholesterol: 0mg	Sodium: 500mg
Vitamin A: 80%	Vitamin C: 120%	Calcium: 8%
Iron: 15%		

Avocado Toast

Prep Time: 5 minutes, **Total Time:** 5 minutes, **Servings:** 2

Ingredients

- 4 slices of whole-grain toast
- 2 ripe avocados, mashed
- Cherry tomatoes, halved
- A sprinkle of nutritional yeast or seeds (e.g., chia, flax, or sesame)

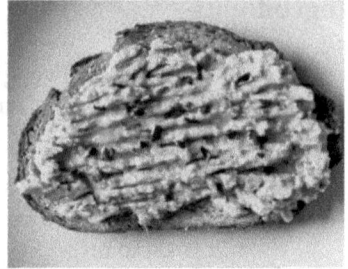

Instructions

1. Toast the whole-grain bread slices until they reach your desired level of crispiness.
2. Spread the mashed avocado evenly onto each toasted slice.
3. Top the avocado toast with halved cherry tomatoes and a sprinkle of your chosen nutritional yeast or seeds.
4. Serve the avocado toast as a nutrient-packed and satisfying lunch option.

Nutritional Information (per serving):

Calories: 250
Fiber: 8g
Saturated Fat: 2g
Vitamin A: 6%
Iron: 6%

Protein: 6g
Sugars: 3g
Cholesterol: 0mg
Vitamin C: 30%

Carbohydrates: 25g
Fat: 15g
Sodium: 150mg
Calcium: 2%

Salmon with Quinoa and Steamed Broccoli

Prep Time: 15 minutes, **Total Time:** 30 minutes, **Servings:** 2

Ingredients

- Baked salmon fillet
- Quinoa (pre-cooked)
- Steamed broccoli with a drizzle of lemon and olive oil

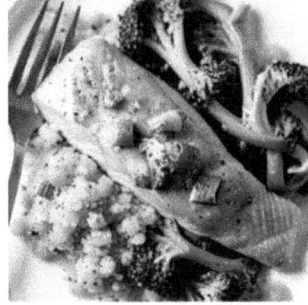

Instructions

1. Prepare the baked salmon fillet as desired. Season it with your favorite herbs and spices.
2. In a bowl, serve the cooked quinoa.
3. Arrange the steamed broccoli on the plate and drizzle it with a touch of fresh lemon juice and olive oil.
4. Place the salmon fillet on top of the quinoa.
5. Enjoy this balanced dinner rich in omega-3 fatty acids, lean protein, and fiber.

Nutritional Information (per serving):

Calories: 400
Fiber: 6g
Saturated Fat: 2g
Vitamin A: 15%
Iron: 20%

Protein: 35g
Sugars: 4g
Cholesterol: 80mg
Vitamin C: 90%

Carbohydrates: 40g
Fat: 12g
Sodium: 200mg
Calcium: 6%

Chickpea and Vegetable Curry

Prep Time: 20 minutes, **Total Time:** 40 minutes, **Servings:** 2

Ingredients

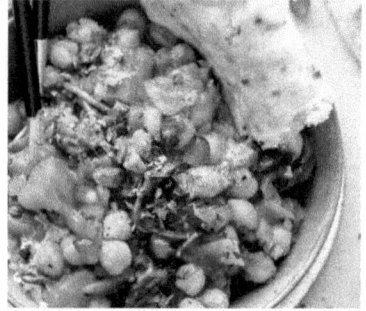

- Chickpeas (canned or cooked)
- A mix of vegetables (e.g., bell peppers, carrots, cauliflower, peas)
- Homemade curry sauce (made from ingredients like coconut milk, curry paste, and spices)
- Brown rice (for serving)

Instructions

1. If using canned chickpeas, rinse and drain them. If using dry chickpeas, cook them according to the package instructions.
2. In a large skillet, stir-fry your choice of vegetables until they are tender.
3. Add the chickpeas and the homemade curry sauce. Stir well and allow it to simmer for a few minutes until the curry is heated through.
4. Serve the chickpea and vegetable curry over brown rice or your grain of choice.
5. Enjoy this flavorful and satisfying dinner, rich in plant-based protein and complex carbohydrates.

Nutritional Information (per serving, without rice):

Calories: 300
Fiber: 10g
Saturated Fat: 1g
Vitamin A: 60%
Iron: 20%

Protein: 12g
Sugars: 8g
Cholesterol: 0mg
Vitamin C: 80%

Carbohydrates: 40g
Fat: 10g
Sodium: 450mg
Calcium: 15%

Baked Sweet Potato with Black Beans

Prep Time: 10 minutes, **Total Time:** 55 minutes, **Servings:** 2

Ingredients

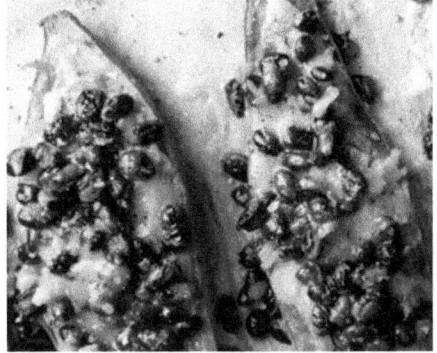

- Baked sweet potatoes
- Black beans (canned or cooked)
- Fresh salsa
- A dollop of Greek yogurt (or a dairy-free alternative)

Instructions

1. Preheat the oven to 400°F (200°C). Wash and scrub the sweet potatoes.
2. Pierce each sweet potato a few times with a fork. Place them on a baking sheet and bake for 45 minutes or until they're soft on the inside.
3. While the sweet potatoes are baking, heat the black beans in a saucepan or microwave until they're warm.
4. Once the sweet potatoes are done, split them open and fluff the flesh with a fork.
5. Top each sweet potato with warmed black beans, fresh salsa, and a dollop of Greek yogurt or a dairy-free alternative.
6. Enjoy this nutrient-packed and comforting dinner that's rich in fiber and protein.

Nutritional Information (per serving):

Calories: 300
Fiber: 12g
Saturated Fat: 1g
Vitamin A: 380%

Protein: 12g
Sugars: 6g
Cholesterol: 5mg
Vitamin C: 25%

Carbohydrates: 50g
Fat: 6g
Sodium: 350mg
Calcium: 15%

Greek Yogurt with Berries

Prep Time: 2 minutes, **Total Time:** 2 minutes, **Servings:** 1

Ingredients

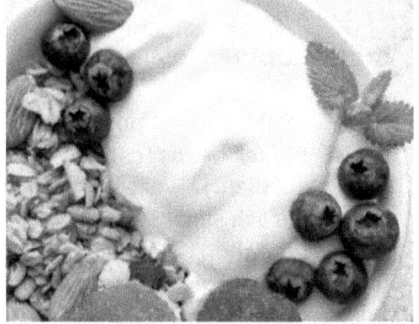

- Greek yogurt
- Fresh berries (e.g., strawberries, blueberries, raspberries)
- A drizzle of honey

Instructions

1. In a bowl, scoop out your desired amount of Greek yogurt.

2. Top the yogurt with a generous serving of fresh berries.

3. Drizzle a touch of honey over the berries for natural sweetness.

4. Stir it all together or enjoy in layers for a visually appealing snack.

5. This snack offers probiotics, antioxidants, and a delightful balance of creaminess and natural sweetness.

Nutritional Information:

Calories: 150
Fiber: 2g
Saturated Fat: 1g
Vitamin A: 6%
Iron: 2%

Protein: 10g
Sugars: 15g
Cholesterol: 10mg
Vitamin C: 15%

Carbohydrates: 20g
Fat: 3g
Sodium: 40mg
Calcium: 15%

Almonds and Dark Chocolate

Prep Time: 1-minute, **Total Time:** 1 minute, **Servings:** 1

Ingredients

- A handful of raw almonds
- A few squares of dark chocolate (70% cocoa or higher)

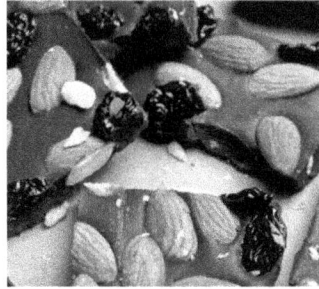

Instructions

1. Measure out a small handful of raw almonds.

2. Pair them with a few squares of dark chocolate (70% cocoa or higher).

3. Enjoy this satisfying combination of healthy fats, protein, and antioxidants.

Nutritional Information:

Calories: 180
Fiber: 3g
Saturated Fat: 3g
Vitamin A: 0%
Iron: 8%

Protein: 4g
Sugars: 5g
Cholesterol: 0mg
Vitamin C: 0%

Carbohydrates: 10g
Fat: 15g
Sodium: 0mg
Calcium: 4%

Sliced Apple with Nut Butter

Prep Time: 5 minutes, **Total Time:** 5 minutes, **Servings:** 1

Ingredients

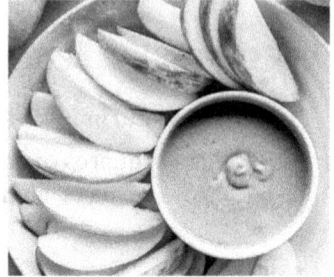

- Sliced apple (e.g., Granny Smith, Fuji)
- Almond or peanut butter

Instructions

1. Wash, core, and slice an apple into wedges or rounds.

2. Pair the apple slices with your choice of almond or peanut butter for dipping.

3. Enjoy this quick and nutritious snack that combines carbohydrates and healthy fats for sustained energy.

Nutritional Information:

Calories: 220	Protein: 5g	Carbohydrates: 25g
Fiber: 6g	Sugars: 18g	Fat: 12g
Saturated Fat: 2g	Cholesterol: 0mg	Sodium: 90mg
Vitamin A: 0%	Vitamin C: 8%	Calcium: 6%
Iron: 6%		

Chapter 12:

Staying Connected to Mind, Body, and Spirit

Your journey toward a holistic lifestyle is not a destination; it is an ongoing, lifelong path. The holistic lifestyle is about making choices every day that nourish and support your overall well-being. In this chapter, we'll explore ways to maintain your connection with your mind, body, and spirit, ensuring that your holistic lifestyle continues to bring lasting well-being and transformation.

Continuing Your Mindfulness and Spiritual Practices

Daily Meditation: Meditation is a powerful tool to maintain a connection with your inner self. Commit to daily meditation, even if it's just for a few minutes. It's during these moments of stillness and introspection that you can find inner peace and heightened self-awareness. As you navigate the inevitable stresses and challenges of life, your meditation practice will help you stay grounded and focused. Whether you prefer guided meditations, breathing exercises, or silent contemplation, your daily meditation will keep your mind, body, and spirit aligned.

Mindful Eating: Mindful eating is a practice that extends the benefits of your detox program into your daily life. Continue savoring each bite of your meals and pay attention to your body's hunger and fullness cues. The habit of mindful eating can promote a healthy and respectful relationship with food. By being fully present during meals, you allow yourself to truly taste and appreciate the nourishment you provide to your body. This practice discourages overeating and emotional eating, as you become attuned to your body's actual needs. A commitment to mindful eating can support your physical and emotional well-being.

Gratitude Journaling: Maintaining your gratitude journal is a simple yet profound practice. Regularly reflecting on the things you're grateful for can significantly enhance your emotional well-being and your overall outlook on life. By consciously acknowledging the blessings, both big and small, you invite positivity and abundance into your life. Gratitude journaling can shift your focus from what you lack to what you have, fostering contentment and a sense of richness in your daily existence. It's a practice that continually reminds you to appreciate life's gifts and remain open to its beauty.

Incorporating these mindfulness and spiritual practices into your daily life requires dedication and commitment. However, the rewards are immeasurable, contributing to lasting well-being, peace, and fulfillment. By nurturing your connection with your mind, body, and spirit, you ensure that your holistic lifestyle is not confined to a short-term program but rather an ongoing journey of growth and transformation.

Deepening Your Connection

Nature Immersion: Nature holds incredible healing and grounding power. Regularly spending time in natural settings, whether it's a walk in the park, hiking in the woods, or simply sitting in your garden, can have profound effects on your well-being. Nature immersion allows you to disconnect from the fast-paced modern world and reconnect with the simplicity and beauty of the natural world. It can be a source of inspiration, serenity, and rejuvenation. The sight of lush greenery, the sound of rustling leaves, and the feeling of fresh air can invigorate your spirit, reduce stress, and provide moments of awe and wonder.

Yoga and Movement: Incorporating yoga or other mindful movement practices into your routine is an excellent way to bridge the gap between your body and mind. Yoga, in particular, emphasizes the connection between physical postures, breath, and mental focus. These practices enhance flexibility, strength, and balance, offering a holistic approach to physical well-being. Engaging in mindful movement is a way to listen to your body and become attuned to its needs. Whether you attend classes or practice at home, yoga and movement can be a space for self-care and a means to maintain harmony between your physical and mental states.

Mindful Relationships: Relationships play a pivotal role in holistic living. Nurturing your connections with others is vital for your overall well-being. One key aspect of mindful relationships is practicing active listening. When you engage in active listening, you are fully present in the conversation, giving your undivided attention to the speaker. This fosters genuine connection and understanding. Empathy is another essential component of mindful relationships. It involves recognizing and acknowledging the emotions and experiences of others, which strengthens your bonds and contributes to a more compassionate and empathetic world. Open communication, characterized by honesty and vulnerability, is yet another facet of mindful relationships. When you communicate openly, you allow your authentic self to be seen, deepening trust and emotional intimacy. These practices can help build a strong support system, nurturing your well-being in times of both joy and challenge.

Deepening your connection with nature, your body, and your relationships is a testament to your commitment to holistic living. By spending time in nature, practicing mindful movement, and fostering mindful relationships, you strengthen your bond with the world around you and the inner world within you. This interplay between the external and internal aspects of your being is where lasting well-being and transformation can flourish.

Stories of Transformation

Real-life stories can be powerful sources of inspiration. Here are a few stories of individuals who have transformed their lives holistically:

Sarah's Mindful Healing: A Journey to Inner Peace

Sarah's story is one of resilience and transformation. For years, she grappled with anxiety that seemed to cast a perpetual shadow over every aspect of her life. The relentless whirlwind of thoughts and worries not only affected her mental health but also took a toll on her physical well-being. Anxiety had become a constant companion, limiting her ability to find peace and happiness.

One fateful day, Sarah decided that she couldn't continue living in the grip of her anxious mind. She sought solace in mindfulness meditation, holding onto a glimmer of hope that it might provide some relief from her inner turmoil. She took the first step on her journey towards healing by dedicating just a few minutes each day to her practice.

In the beginning, it was challenging. Sarah struggled to quiet the persistent chatter of her anxious thoughts. However, she persevered, each day returning to her practice, focusing on her breath, and learning to be fully present in the moment. She gradually started to understand that the present moment was a sanctuary from the turmoil of her mind.

Over time, something remarkable began to happen. Sarah noticed a significant reduction in her anxiety levels. It was as though the practice of mindfulness was helping her unravel the tightly wound threads of anxiety that had bound her for so long. She found a newfound sense of clarity and calm that had eluded her for years. As her mindfulness practice deepened, she discovered the power of self-compassion, allowing her to be kind and patient with herself as she navigated her journey to inner peace.

Sarah's transformation was not instantaneous, but it was profound. The daily commitment and consistency of her mindfulness practice played a pivotal role in her healing. With each passing day, she felt more empowered to respond to life's challenges with resilience and grace.

Sarah's journey serves as a poignant reminder of the profound impact that even small daily practices can have on our overall well-being. It underscores the transformative potential that lies within our commitment to healing and self-improvement. Sarah's story is a testament to the resilience of the human spirit and the boundless capacity for positive change to find inner peace and well-being.

Mark's Plant-Based Transformation: A Journey to Vitality

Mark's journey is a remarkable testament to the transformative power of dietary choices. For many years, Mark was a dedicated omnivore, savoring hearty meat-based meals with an unbridled love for the flavors and traditions of his cuisine. He reveled in the sensory experience of every bite, cherishing the rich and savory tastes that graced his plate. However, a lingering sense of sluggishness and excess weight gnawed at him, whispering a need for change.

One day, Mark decided to begin an experiment that would forever alter the course of his life: he would transition to a plant-based diet for just one month. This decision marked the beginning of a journey to holistic well-being that he had never imagined.

The results of Mark's experiment were nothing short of astonishing. Almost immediately, he felt a surge in his energy levels that seemed to defy explanation. The feeling of perpetual sluggishness began to lift, and he felt lighter, both physically and mentally. It was as though his body had found a renewed sense of vitality. His palate began to appreciate the myriad flavors and textures that plant-based foods offered, and he realized that he didn't need meat to satisfy his culinary desires.

The positive effects of this dietary shift didn't stop at increased energy. As the weeks passed, Mark noticed the number on the scale gradually decreasing. Those extra pounds he had carried for so long seemed to melt away. He felt more agile, more in tune with his body, and more comfortable in his skin than he had in years.

However, it wasn't just Mark's physical health that was undergoing a significant transformation. His mental clarity soared to new heights, and a sense of overall well-being washed over him. He felt more connected to the world around him, appreciating not only the nourishment he provided his body but also the positive impact of his dietary choices on the environment.

Mark's month-long experiment had revealed a profound truth: that the food we consume has a direct and powerful impact on our physical and mental well-being. This realization was life-altering. Mark decided that he wouldn't return to his previous eating habits; instead, he chose to embrace a predominantly plant-based diet as his new way of life.

Today, Mark thrives on a diet primarily composed of plant-based foods, and he enjoys not only the physical benefits but also the heightened mental clarity and sense of well-being that accompany his choices. His journey showcases how even a short experiment with holistic living can lead to profound, life-altering transformations. It underscores the idea that a single conscious choice can set the course for a life of well-being and vitality.

Ella's Spiritual Awakening: A Journey to Inner Peace and Purpose

Ella's life was a tapestry woven with an insatiable yearning for something deeper and more meaningful. From her earliest memories, she had always felt a pull toward the ineffable, a yearning to explore the spiritual dimensions of existence that existed beyond the surface of daily life. This quest for purpose and understanding was the compass that guided her journey into the realm of holistic living.

Ella's spiritual journey was a meandering path, marked by exploration and contemplation. She delved into various faiths and spiritual practices, seeking the resonance of truth that would harmonize with her heart and soul. In her quest, she attended places of worship, engaged in meditation and prayer, and explored the profound teachings of spiritual leaders throughout history. With each step, Ella's connection with the spiritual dimension deepened, and her understanding of her place in the universe expanded.

Over time, Ella discovered a spiritual path that resonated with her on the deepest levels. It was as if she had found a missing piece of a grand puzzle, and the sense of clarity and peace it brought her was akin to finding a long-lost treasure. This spiritual awakening was not just a change in her beliefs; it was a transformation of her entire being. She felt a profound sense of purpose that had eluded her for much of her life. The tumultuous waves of restlessness and uncertainty that had once defined her existence were replaced by a serene inner peace.

Ella's story is a powerful testament to the idea that the spiritual dimension of holistic living is not a destination but a journey, a lifelong pilgrimage of self-discovery and exploration. It emphasizes that spirituality is a deeply personal and subjective experience that cannot be standardized or prescribed. Ella's journey underlines the transformative power of seeking and aligning with one's deeper purpose.

In many ways, Ella's journey reflects the profound truth that when we explore the spiritual dimension of our existence, we awaken to a deeper sense of purpose and meaning. Her story is a reminder that everyone's spiritual journey is unique and should be embraced without judgment or preconceived notions. Ella's spiritual awakening stands as a testament to the idea that when we connect with our inner selves and seek the profound truths of existence, we unlock the transformative power of holistic living.

These stories exemplify the transformative power of holistic living. They underscore the significance of staying connected to your mind, body, and spirit, and how it can lead to continued growth and vitality. Remember that your path to holistic living is personal and adaptable, tailored to your individual needs and preferences. By cultivating mindfulness, engaging in spiritual practices, and committing to holistic well-being, you can experience ongoing transformation and lasting well-being.

Chapter 12:
Your Holistic Journey Continues

As we conclude this journey towards holistic well-being, it's essential to reflect on the key takeaways from this book and to encourage you to continue a lifelong path of holistic living.

Key Takeaways:

Holistic Living Is an Ongoing Journey: Holistic well-being is not a destination but a lifelong journey. It's about continuously nurturing and balancing your physical, mental, emotional, and spiritual aspects.

- **Mindfulness and Connection:** Daily practices like meditation, mindful eating, and gratitude journaling can keep you grounded and connected to yourself.

- **Nourishing Your Body:** The recipes provided in this book are a gateway to nourishing your body with wholesome and nutritious ingredients. Eating well is a fundamental part of holistic living.

- **Physical Activity**: Regular exercise, whether it's yoga, hiking, or any other movement practice, connects your body and mind while promoting strength and flexibility.

- **Healthy Relationships:** Mindful relationships characterized by active listening, empathy, and open communication are vital for your holistic well-being.

- **Personalized Holistic Journey:** Your holistic journey is unique to you. It should adapt to your needs and preferences. There's no one-size-fits-all approach to holistic living.

- **Stories of Transformation:** The inspirational stories of Sarah's mindful healing, Mark's plant-based transformation, and Ella's spiritual awakening illustrate the profound effects holistic living can have on your life.

Now that you've gained insight into holistic living, I encourage you to begin or continue your journey towards a more vibrant, healthier, and balanced you. Remember that it's not about perfection but progress. Take small steps each day to align with your holistic well-being goals.

Remember, your holistic journey is a lifelong endeavor that encompasses your mind, body, and spirit. Continue to explore, learn, and grow on this path. The more you invest in your well-being, the richer and more fulfilling your life will become. Embrace the journey and thrive in holistic living!

Appendices

Appendix A: Detox Program Journal

Appendix B: Mindfulness and Meditation Resources

Appendix C: Holistic Recipe Index

Detox Program Journal

14-Day Detox Program Journal

Program Start Date: _____

Program End Date: _____

Day 1: Date - _____

Morning Reflection:
- Mood:

- Energy Level:

- Physical Symptoms (if any):

- Morning Affirmation or Intention:

Daily Nutrition:
- Breakfast:

- Lunch:

- Dinner:

- Snacks:

- Hydration (Water, Herbal Tea, etc.):

Physical Activity:
- Type and Duration:

Mindfulness and Meditation:
- Practice Details (e.g., meditation, mindful breathing):

- Emotional Well-being:

Emotions Experienced:
- Stressors:

- Coping Strategies:

Evening Reflection:
- Mood:

- Energy Level:

- Physical Symptoms (if any):

- Evening Affirmation or Intention:

Day 2: Date - _____

Morning Reflection:
- Mood:

- Energy Level:

- Physical Symptoms (if any):

- Morning Affirmation or Intention:

Daily Nutrition:

- Breakfast:

- Lunch:

- Dinner:

- Snacks:

- Hydration (Water, Herbal Tea, etc.):

Physical Activity:
- Type and Duration:

Mindfulness and Meditation:
- Practice Details (e.g., meditation, mindful breathing):

Emotional Well-being:
- Emotions Experienced:

- Stressors:

- Coping Strategies:

Evening Reflection:
- Mood:

- Energy Level:

- Physical Symptoms (if any):

- Evening Affirmation or Intention:

Continue daily entries for the next 12 days.

Morning Reflection:
- Mood:

- Energy Level:

- Physical Symptoms (if any):

- Morning Affirmation or Intention:

Daily Nutrition:
- Breakfast:

- Lunch:

- Dinner:

- Snacks:

- Hydration (Water, Herbal Tea, etc.):

Physical Activity:
- Type and Duration:

Mindfulness and Meditation:
- Practice Details (e.g., meditation, mindful breathing):

Emotional Well-being:
- Emotions Experienced:

- Stressors:

- Coping Strategies:

Evening Reflection:
- Mood:

- Energy Level:

- Physical Symptoms (if any):

- Evening Affirmation or Intention:

Program End Date: _____

Congratulations on completing your 14-Day Detox Program! Your holistic well-being journey continues.

Appendix B:
Mindfulness and Meditation Resources

Recommended Books:

- "The Miracle of Mindfulness" by Thich Nhat Hanh

- "Wherever You Go, There You Are" by Jon Kabat-Zinn

- "Radical Acceptance" by Tara Brach

- "The Power of Now" by Eckhart Tolle

- "10% Happier" by Dan Harris

Recommended Apps:

- Headspace

- Calm

- Insight Timer

- Waking Up with Sam Harris

- Buddhify

Websites for Further Resources:

- Mindful.org

- Greater Good Science Center

- Mindfulness Exercises

- Tara Brach's Guided Meditations

Appendix C:
Holistic Recipe Index

This index provides easy reference to the recipes featured in this book, categorized by meal type.

Breakfast Recipes:

Green Smoothie Bowl

- Page Number: 65
- Ingredients: spinach, banana, almond milk, chia seeds, mixed berries, granola

Chia Pudding

- Page Number: 66
- Ingredients: chia seeds, almond milk, honey, fresh fruit

Overnight Oats

- Page Number: 68
- Ingredients: rolled oats, almond milk, Greek yogurt, honey, mixed berries

Lunch Recipes:

Quinoa Salad

- Page Number: 69

- Ingredients: quinoa, cucumber, cherry tomatoes, bell peppers, fresh herbs, lemon-tahini dressing

Vegetable Stir-Fry

- Page Number: 70

- Ingredients: mixed veggies, tofu or tempeh, homemade stir-fry sauce

Avocado Toast

- Page Number: 72

- Ingredients: whole-grain toast, mashed avocado, cherry tomatoes, nutritional yeast, or seeds

---

Dinner Recipes:

Salmon with Quinoa and Steamed Broccoli

- Page Number: 74

- Ingredients: baked salmon fillet, quinoa, steamed broccoli with lemon and olive oil

Chickpea and Vegetable Curry

- Page Number: 75

- Ingredients: chickpeas, assorted veggies, homemade curry sauce, served with brown rice

Baked Sweet Potato with Black Beans

- Page Number: 77

- Ingredients: baked sweet potato, black beans, fresh salsa, Greek yogurt

---

Snack Ideas:

Greek Yogurt with Berries

- Page Number: 78

- Ingredients: Greek yogurt, fresh berries, honey

Almonds and Dark Chocolate

- Page Number: 80

- Ingredients: raw almonds, dark chocolate squares (70% cocoa or higher)

Sliced Apple with Nut Butter

- Page Number: 81

- Ingredients: apple slices, almond or peanut butter

www.ingramcontent.com/pod-product-compliance
Lightning Source LLC
Chambersburg PA
CBHW060225030426
42335CB00014B/1344